Transformational
HEALING

Free yourself from fatigue, digestive issues, thyroid dysfunction, stress, and autoimmune

Kirstin Carey, CHN, NLPP, CBTP, CTP, BHIP, Chef
Anthony DiNobile, BCHN, CFBCA, MMS, CNM, CPT

DOWNLOAD THE COMPANION GUIDEBOOK FOR FREE!

To say thanks for getting a copy of our book, we would like to give you the Transformational Healing guidebook for FREE!

We know you're more likely to get the most out of this book if you have the companion guidebook. We created it so you can move through the exercises and customize them to your needs.

Instead of paying $10-$20 for the guidebook, we'd like to give it to you for free...

Just click on the QR Code below with your phone camera, or go directly to **www.nourish123.com/thbonus**

You'll see this QR code throughout the book, indicating where you can use the Guidebook to deepen your learning.

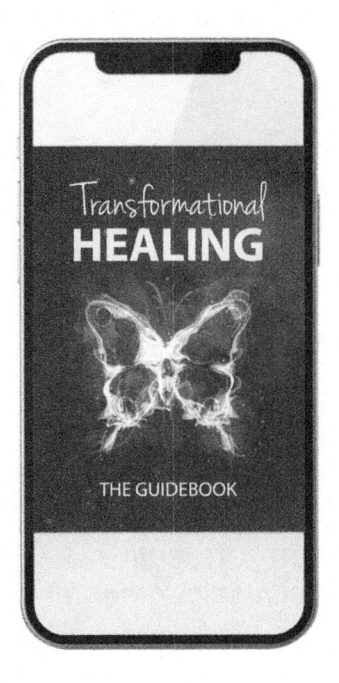

SCAN ME!

WANT A VIDEO SUMMARY OF THIS BOOK?

Get a quick video summary of this book that guides you through the proven system of transformational healing.

Watch now as we take you through the visual presentation of all the necessary components to finding your unique healing path. Make sure to get your notebook and colorful pens ready!

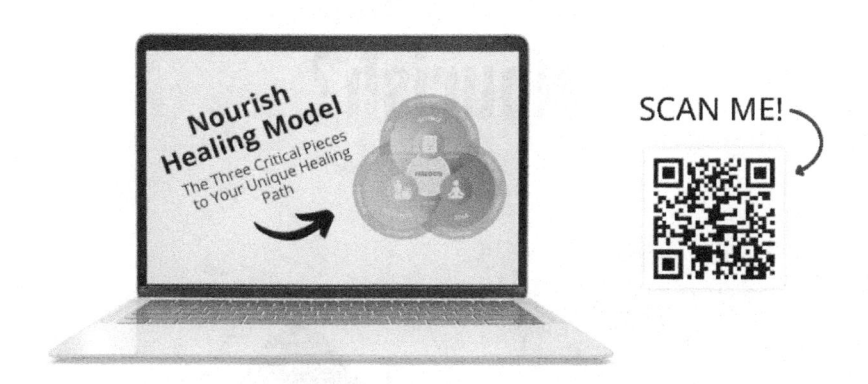

In this video, we cover 3 things:

1. The Proven Process to finding your unique healing path
2. How to identify the missing pieces in your puzzle
3. How to successfully take next steps towards filling in the gaps

Scan QR code to access this video or go to www.nourish123.com/thbonus!

Want Our Help at
Nourish?

Want our help implementing the content in this book?

At Nourish, our goal is to save you 100's of hours and 1,000's of dollars in the process... and to help you get on your unique healing journey so you experience the life you want.

If you want to go further faster with your health and you're serious about getting our help, book a call with the team to put together a plan and see how we can help.

www.nourish123.com/heal

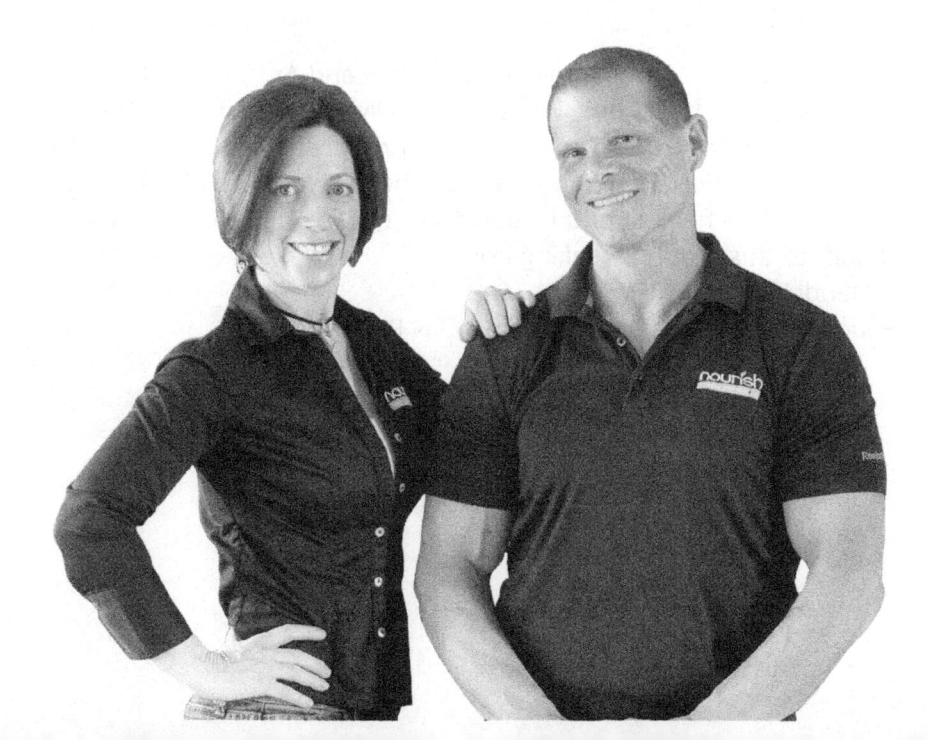

ENDORSEMENTS:

"Kind Hearts, Fierce Minds, Strong Spirits. Kirstin and Anthony are the real thing. Read this book and take a quantum leap into your best life."
~ Dr. Beverley Dowdell, ND, MA CANTAB
Cambridge University

"A MUST read for anyone interested in health as a functional holistic experience or who wants to transform personally! The authors brilliantly debunk the traditional pathological and mechanist health model. Kirstin and Anthony show extraordinary healing in everyday people by dynamically using science, nutrition, and inner soul work. They have woven the scientific teachings of *Breaking the Habit of Being You,* the therapeutic knowledge of *The Myth of Normal,* and somatic wisdom of *The Body Keeps Score* into one usable, applicable, easy-to-read book anyone can use to eliminate symptoms and heal. Life changing for my own health. This will be a required reading for all my coaching clients! "
~ Dr. Lori C. Ebert
Health Educator and Relationship & Sexual Wellness Coach
www.DrLoriEbert.com

"Wow, what a liberating book! Kirstin Carey and Anthony DiNobile pull back the curtain on what is really required for healing. Transformational Healing gives us comprehensive practical tools that are backed by science and help us grow in ways we never thought possible. True healing and freedom are now within everyone's reach, thanks to this groundbreaking book."
~ Mahdi Brown, NMD
Founder & Managing Director of OKAN Resilience Ltd.

Copyright (c) 2023 Kirstin Carey, Anthony DiNobile.
All rights reserved.

Published by Butterfly Books, Inc.: www.ButterflyBooks123.com

No part of this publication may be reproduced, distributed, or transmitted in any form or by any means, including photocopying, recording, or other electronic or mechanical methods, without the prior written permission of the publisher, except in the case of brief quotations embodied in reviews and certain other non-commercial uses permitted by copyright law.

The authors of this book do not dispense medical advice or prescribe the use of any technique as a form of treatment for physical, emotional, or medical problems without the advice of a physician, either directly or indirectly. The intent of the author is to only offer information of a general nature to help you in your quest for emotional, physical, or spiritual well-being. In the event you use any of the information in this book for yourself, the author and publisher assume no responsibility for your actions.

Cataloging-in-Publication Data is on file as the Library of Congress.

Print ISBN: 979-8-218-02175-7
E-book ISBN: 979-8-218-02176-4
Audiobook ISBN:

DEDICATION

This book is dedicated to everyone looking for answers to feeling healthy, whole, and free from the chains of inflammation. Your symptoms or diagnosis don't have to control your story. Listen to the voice in your soul saying you can live the life you want.

Because you can.

TABLE OF CONTENTS

OPENING: THE EVERYDAY MIRACLE	1
PART 1: CLARITY	11
CHAPTER 1: GOALS	13
CHAPTER 2: SYMPTOMS	19
CHAPTER 3: TIMELINE	23
CHAPTER 4: TRIGGERS, TRAUMAS, AND BLOCKS	29
CHAPTER 5: SELF ATTACK	33
CHAPTER 6 HIDDEN DRIVERS	37
CHAPTER 7: WHAT IS (NEGATIVE) TRAUMA?	41
CHAPTER 8: BLOCKS ARE THERE TO KEEP YOU SAFE	45
PART 2: NUTRITION	49
CHAPTER 9: FOOD	51
CHAPTER 10: SUPPLEMENTS	59
CHAPTER 11: MOVEMENT	63
CHAPTER 12: SLEEP	69
PART 3: SCIENCE	71
CHAPTER 13: ADRENAL FUNCTION	73
CHAPTER 14: THE IMMUNE SYSTEM	79
CHAPTER 15: LABS	85
CHAPTER 16: PHYSIOLOGY	91
CHAPTER 17: MEDICATION	99
CHAPTER 18: EPIGENETICS	107
PART 4: SOUL	117
CHAPTER 19: THE FRACTURED SOUL	119
CHAPTER 20: WHAT'S YOUR PURPOSE	123
CHAPTER 21: IDENTITY	129
CHAPTER 22: PARADIGM & BELIEF	139

CHAPTER 23: NEGATIVE VS POSITIVE TRAUMA 143

CHAPTER 24: WOUNDED CHILDREN 147

CHAPTER 25: SYMPTOMS ARE A MESSAGE 153

CHAPTER 26: INTERPRETING SYMPTOMS 161

CHAPTER 27: YOUR FILTER & FAMILIAR PATTERNS 165

CHAPTER 28: YOUR PARADIGM ISN'T LOGICAL (AND NEITHER ARE YOU) ...169

PART 5: THE PLAN 173

CHAPTER 29: IDENTIFYING HURDLES HEALING 175

CHAPTER 30: DEFENSE MECHANISMS 179

CHAPTER 31: CHANGING YOUR TRAJECTORY 189

CHAPTER 32: THREE KINDS OF PEOPLE 201

END: TAKING ACTION AND FINDING YOUR FREEDOM 205

ENDNOTES 208

FORWARD

In May 2020, I started a quest to find and interview experts in the health and wellness arena who were doing something different, who were changing lives and who were looking "outside the box." I was introduced to Kirstin and Anthony by one of their fellow colleagues, a naturopath in Europe, Dr. Mahdi. When he told me that you could reverse autoimmune disease and that Kirstin and Anthony guided people through this process, my interest was piqued!

At the time, I just wanted to interview both of them for my Weekend Wellness Hour Show to share this incredible information with others. Little did I know that I would be relying on them to help me through my own health challenge a few months later.

My own work as founder of the PABR® Institute includes guiding clients through a process to calm down the fight or flight nervous system to alleviate pain, stress, anxiety, insomnia and the need for various orthopedic surgeries. This process works great and helps countless people all over the world, but most people need help and guidance in multiple areas to rebuild their health.

Kirstin and Anthony provide that comprehensive approach that most people need for their health, especially when it comes to autoimmune conditions. They have a system that helps you examine not only the nutritional and chemical part of your health but also the spiritual side. Their book, Transformational Healing, gives you excellent written guidance on how to start examining your own health.

Why not just go to a doctor and get pills and/or invasive procedures? Why become responsible for your own healing? Here's a personal example that I alluded to earlier.

In June 2020, I became sick with COVID after a business trip to Belize and I had a high fever for 10 days (102-103 degrees). I dropped 10 lbs in a week and was very ill. My immune system did its job and I recovered well, but some of my circulating hormones and organ systems were a bit off. I noticed it when my hair began to fall out….in clumps.

I had thin curly hair to begin with, but from July to November, I lost 90% of my hair and had bald spots all over. While we all say that appearances don't or shouldn't matter, the truth is that they do, especially in the health and wellness space where we look at the outward appearance of a person to determine how healthy he or she is based on his or her habits.

This hair loss was very embarrassing and devastating since I was in the public eye speaking at events, speaking on my livestream show and working with clients visually on Zoom. I didn't know what to do and didn't want more chemicals in my body from the various hair regrowth solutions (especially since my beliefs about healing stem from what we have inside us), but Kirstin and Anthony stepped up and offered help.

Anthony looked at my bloodwork and although it looked almost normal according to the "norms," he saw deficiencies that were created from being ill for 10 days. I began to address them immediately through targeted organic foods. Within a few weeks, I started to see some hair regrowth. My body was responding well to adjusting my nutrition to make sure I had the correct nutrients to support my organ systems. I have since worked with Kirstin on releasing blocks in my body and soul so that my body feels more connected with all its parts and there is a flow.

My example is just one of many who have benefited from Kirstin and Anthony. Mine was mild and a relatively quick fix that took several months versus some of their clients who have had autoimmune conditions for decades. It's truly powerful to see those with much worse conditions shift their healing and learn to thrive again.

There is so much to health. Having the correct support team and resources to guide you through what creates health for YOU is vital. Each person, including their past experiences, their present body, and their future desires creates a unique ecosystem inside himself or herself with a certain needs. Kirstin and Anthony are genuine, authentic, caring guides who continually provide the latest information in healing. Their knowledge of healing is unsurpassed.

As you work your way through this book, I suggest pausing at the beginning to take note of your current health state. Look at all aspects so that you can see how far you transform in the healing journey that Kirstin and Anthony take you on. You have made an excellent choice in guides.

Dr Amy Novotny
Founder of PABR® Institute, Entrepreneur, Doctor of PT, Breathing/Pain Specialist, Speaker, Author, Ultra Marathoner, Award-winning Photographer

If not now, when?

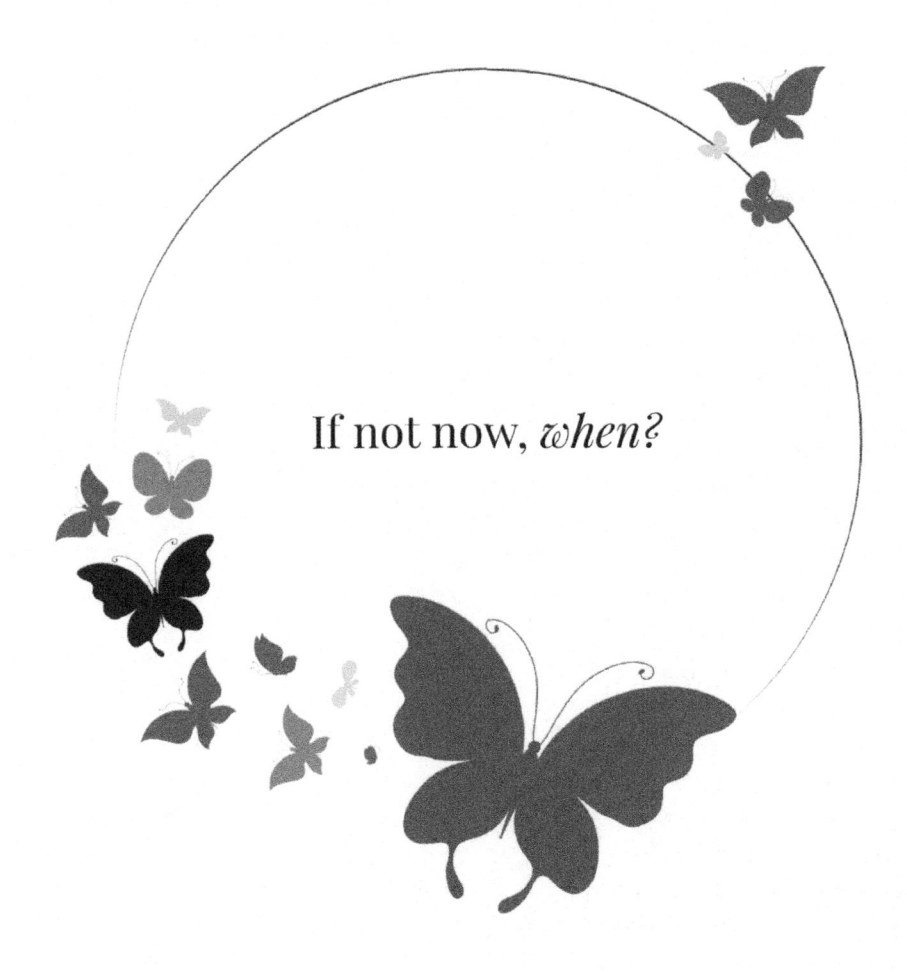

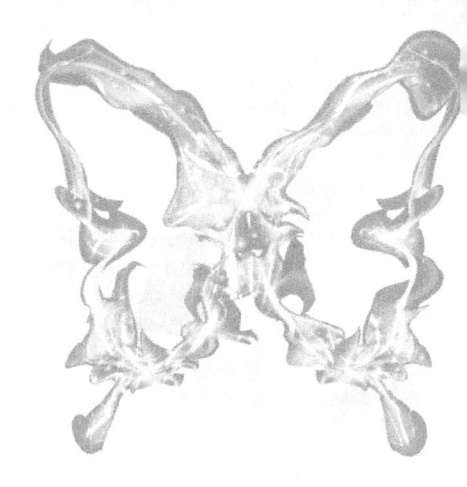

OPENING:

THE EVERYDAY MIRACLE

Meghan was 41 years old when she contacted our office several years ago to see if we could help her with her overactive thyroid. She had been diagnosed with Graves' disease, and was struggling with symptoms such as inability to gain weight, brain fog, muscle loss, low self-confidence, irritability, anxiety, hair loss, sleeplessness, racing heart, and palpitations. She was exhausted and felt like she was always "late for something" even when she had nothing scheduled.

Hours after Meghan enrolled in our program, she called in a panic.

"My doctor just called. He told me if I 'didn't remove my thyroid immediately' I would 'suffer and die!' He wants to schedule surgery for Monday. What do I do?"

Based on Meghan's most recent labs, her thyroid was out of control. Her immune system was attacking her thyroid causing it to go into "hyper" mode. Her doctor had never seen anyone heal their thyroid. His only experience with overactive or under-active thyroid was to forcibly "correct it" with medication or surgery. The drawbacks to either of these recommendations were a myriad of side effects. And with the surgery option, there was no going back once the gland was removed. Her body would be dependent on medication and she would have to deal with the side effects for the rest of her life.

We discussed the various options with Meghan, but, of course, she ultimately had to make the decision on what to do. She was understandably frightened. It would be a life-changing decision.

Meghan chose to push the surgery option off, despite her doctor insisting she was making a literally fatal mistake, and see what progress she could make addressing her physical and emotional stressors. We created a plan for her to address her nutrition and support her adrenal function (which is directly connected to thyroid function), ran some additional tests to better understand her gut imbalances, and worked with her on processing her stress response more effectively. Meghan, like most of us, had underlying traumas and stress that her body was mismanaging, which was keeping her in a constant state of fight-or-flight. This was a large part of the reason her body had been triggered into attack mode.

Within 12 weeks, her thyroid response had calmed down dramatically, and she was feeling in control of her life again. We continued to work with her on her nutrition and stress management.

A little over a year later, Meghan's endocrinologist (the same one who demanded she "remove her thyroid immediately") ran a thyroid lab panel. Here's the email Meghan sent to Anthony after her discussion with her doctor about the lab results.

Hi Anthony! I wanted to share this with you, because no one will appreciate it as much! My endocrinologist finally called me, just talked to him for 20 minutes (way longer than any doctor gives!) and he could not stop telling me he can't believe it!! He has to know what pill I am taking, who is giving me something! I kept saying, Nothing, I promise; it's all been food and treating myself kind!! It went back and forth, and he would NOT believe me! Then he said I need to write a book because people need to know there is another way! Haha that proves how sheltered doctors are, as this way of healing has been written many, many times forever. Haha! Anyway, it was very gratifying!!!

Thanks, Anthony ☺

Meghan's story is awesome, right?

And though Meghan didn't write a book about her experience, we thought it was only fitting to begin this book with her story. Because, she's correct: despite the thousands of others all around the world who have healed from thyroid disorder, heart disease, cancer, IBS, arthritis, gout, anxiety, diabetes, autoimmune, and other issues, most practitioners aren't trained how to help patients find their path to achieve transformational healing.

Meghan's results are not a miracle. But *our bodies* are miracles that were beautifully designed with the inherent ability to heal once they are given the right tools and support.

Healing from symptoms, autoimmune, and chronic illness is possible and not in a "pray for a miracle" kind of way. Symptoms and illness can be reversed and don't need to be lifelong issues. So why oh why do we keep getting told that healing is impossible?

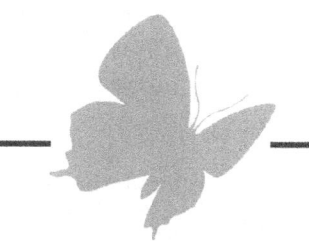

> "Our bodies are miracles that were beautifully designed with the inherent ability to heal once they are given the right tools and support."

Part of the reason is because too many practitioners and doctors don't even realize healing is a possibility because they are focused on "sick management." You don't want to simply manage your symptoms. You want to get to the root cause of them and correct the underlying imbalance creating them.

Just go to our website and see the success stories. Their successes are not accidents. They are not one-in-a-million type miracles. They are examples of how the body WORKS when given the right tools, environment, and support - and when the patient and *the practitioner* both know it's possible.

If you're working with a doctor or practitioner who tells you that you can't heal and that you have to have radical surgeries or take medications for the rest of your life, do yourself a favor and, at least, get a second opinion. Make sure to get an opinion from someone who not only knows it's possible to heal, but someone who has clients who (and perhaps even they themselves) have healed from something similar to what you are going through.

In Chapter 22: Paradigm and Belief, we're going to discuss The Pygmalion Effect, which was discovered by a series of scientific studies of doctors, patients, medications, teachers, and students and the impact belief has on results of healing and learning. The results are fascinating and will help you realize how influential your belief and the belief of others may have on your health and life trajectory.

You must believe there is a way to heal from whatever health challenge you are struggling with right now. Guaranteed there is at least a sliver of belief in your core that knows it's possible for you to find healing or you wouldn't be reading this book.

And that belief, the knowing that your body was designed to heal given the right tools and support, is the powerful core to getting everything you want.

Freedom is the Goal

Do you want transformational healing and to reach true freedom?

Before you answer, let's discuss what "transformational healing" really means and what it takes to achieve it.

Perhaps you've been through other treatments or programs before, and they haven't worked. Or maybe they worked, but it was only for a short period of time.

During that "honeymoon period" of a few days, weeks, or months, you may have felt like things were working, but then you found yourself sliding. Or perhaps you felt even worse than before you started the new restrictive diet, functional nutrition protocol, regimen of supplements, or loads of lab tests.

This often happens because you were promised that in one magic pill, with an easy seven-day detox, doing a three-week diet reset, or some special eight-week health program, you could clear decades of trauma and abuse, underlying emotional patterns, and physical damage.

Essentially, you were told there was an easy or fast way to heal.

Let's get clear: That's not true.

If there were an easy, cheap, fast, comfortable way to heal decades of damage, no one would be sick, right? But in order to truly heal, you have to change in some way, and change can often feel like the hardest thing you can do in your life.

In this book, we are going to show you where to look to know what kind of change needs to be made and how to make those changes for long-term success, and not just feel better temporarily for a couple of days or a few weeks.

True long-term healing, when done correctly and customized to you specifically, eliminates symptoms and reverses disease so you can truly heal.

Here's another truth bomb:

If you have an autoimmune condition, cancer, or other chronic illness, the seed at the very root of your symptoms has been growing for at least a decade or more.

Symptoms, illness, and disease don't just pop up with no warning. They don't just appear one day. They circulate in your system for many years, giving many signals before they present dramatically enough to warrant a diagnosis.

Up to this point, whether you've noticed them or not, you've been receiving signs and messages that there was a problem brewing and something was out of balance emotionally, mentally, or physically.

Here's the big kicker: whatever the original seed was, it's impacting you physically, mentally, and emotionally. All three are always involved because they are intertwined.

When the seed first begins to grow, the warning signs are typically small ones. They are gentle, little nudges from your system alerting you that a shift needs to be made in your thoughts, feelings, or actions.

But over time, if the gentle nudging is ignored, and that underlying root cause isn't addressed, the body increases its attempt to get your attention and bring awareness to the imbalance that's going on.

These nudges could be a headache, fatigue, anxiety, increasing belly fat, or irregular periods. They can also appear as nagging repetitive thoughts, bloating and gas, joint pain, panic attacks, or a hypersensitivity to noises, smells, and chemicals.

For many, the symptoms have to be really dramatic in order to cause awareness.

If you're a high achiever, a "type A" personality, or someone who is good at "white knuckling" it and pushing through, then you're most likely dealing with symptoms that are quite dramatic. But you've been pushing them off, thinking you'll "get through it," which is sending a message to your body that you aren't listening.

When you do that for too long, then the diagnosis for autoimmune disease, cancer, and other chronic illness begins.

And that's not okay.

Our bodies were *designed to heal.*

No matter what you've been told to this point, or how long you've been suffering, be clear: You are not broken. You are 100% capable of healing. You just need to know how to activate your inherent power to heal.

> "You are not broken. You are 100% capable of healing. You just need to know how to activate your inherent power to heal."

Throughout this book, we are going to give you truthful answers on achieving optimal long-term health. Not just the short-term, temporary fixes. And we're going to present you with real answers to eliminate the feelings of being stuck, sick, frustrated, exhausted, out of sorts, or just plain disconnected from knowing who you really are.

We're going to pull apart our proven process and give you details about how we have guided hundreds of people in getting out of crisis and into healing so they could live healthy, happy, and full lives.

Nourish Healing Model

Though we will dissect this model in more depth throughout this book, what you need to understand now is that there are three major components critical to the healing process:

1. Nutrition

2. Science

3. Soul

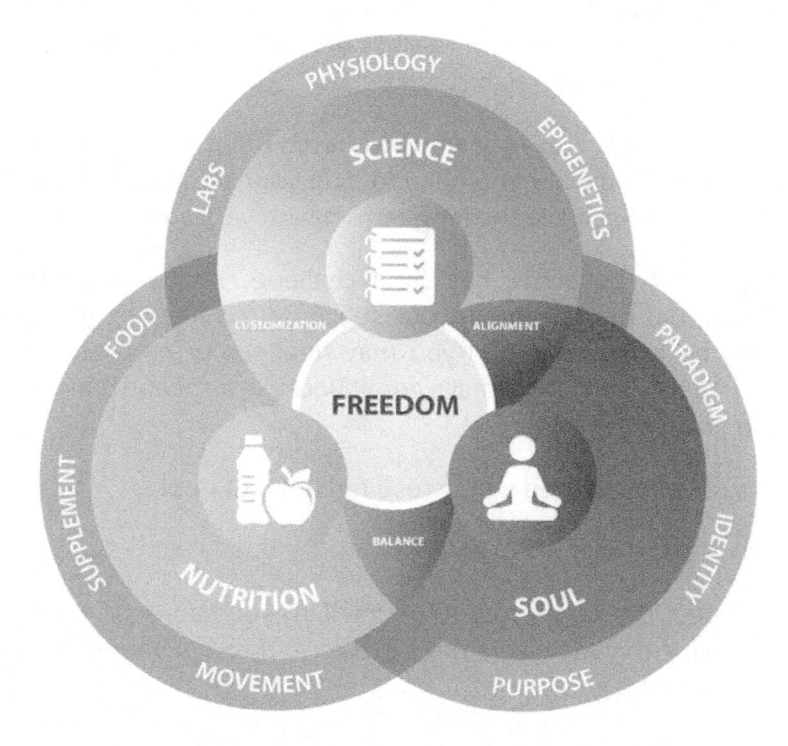

These three pieces must work together cohesively and not against each other. What we have found is that even when people thought they had all of the pieces, if they were experiencing symptoms and disease, then those pieces didn't fit together in a way that created a complete healing solution *for them.*

The nutrition, science, and soul have to dance together synergistically in order to achieve true optimal health. You cannot get the health you want if you are missing any of these pieces.

We're also going to show you how and why past attempts you've made to heal have failed you. You'll gain a much clearer picture of our proven healing process and how to use it to reach your personal health goals.

Specific exercises, processes, and modalities we use with our clients to achieve healing will be revealed for you to gain a deeper understanding of what is blocking your health success and what to do to dissolve those blocks.

We're going to be super honest, sometimes brutally so. Anthony is originally from New York, and Kirstin's originally from Philly; so, we're going to give it to you straight.

We're going to reveal exactly why you haven't found the solution you are looking for and what you need to stop your symptoms, heal from the damage, and achieve the long-term health you want.

We're going to poke the bear and challenge some long-standing paradigms that may hiding in your subconscious keeping you stuck. This may be frustrating, and you may "feel some feels" as you get further into this book. And that's good! Because it means that you are going to finally get answers!

If you're up for that, then you're reading the right book!

So, let's do this thing!

Get centered. Get connected to yourself so you can hear what your body is saying to you. Take a deep breath in through your nose... and open up and let it go.

Now...

Do you want transformational healing?

Why We Wrote This Book

Before we dive straight in, it's important you understand why we wrote this book and what drove us to become natural health practitioners.

Kirstin and Anthony met near the end of 2008 on Match.com. They were each recovering from a divorce. Kirstin, originally from Philadelphia, was a recent transplant to Arizona, and Anthony had moved from New York to the Phoenix area several years before.

Kirstin was a business and marketing consultant and struggled with migraines, allergy attacks, hormone imbalance, acne, digestive issues, rashes, foggy brain, and weight fluctuation. She didn't know it at the time, but she had celiac disease and would later be diagnosed with Hashimoto's.

Anthony was an IT professional at a large law firm, who had been body building since he was 16 years old and had a passion for riding motorcycles, Ducati specifically.

The two hit it off right away but had no idea what a powerful shift the relationship was going to create.

Kirstin continued to struggle with symptoms and saw all the traditional doctors and specialists. She endured all the tests, invasive scopes, and awkward exams. She followed all the recommendations and took the medications as prescribed. She was the perfect patient, except she wasn't getting better. Doctors didn't have any answers for her. They said things like, "Well, I can prescribe you a medication for anxiety. That might help." This, of course, was frustrating because she wasn't anxious. **Something was wrong,** and it was becoming depressing because the experts who were supposed to know how to figure out what was wrong were dismissive.

Kirstin changed her approach and tried to find answers through natural medicine. After spending about $25,000 out-of-pocket, she was diagnosed with celiac disease, an autoimmune condition where the immune system attacks the villi and microvilli in the gut. She was advised to avoid gluten and to take supplements that cost hundreds of dollars a month. Though she did feel somewhat better after eliminating gluten, she knew there still had to be more to the story.

Anthony was frustrated for Kirstin because he didn't know how to help her or best support her during this search, but he did the best he could. Being a bodybuilder for so many years, he understood restrictive diets, but it's hard to understand what someone with autoimmune disease goes through or how to best support them.

In an effort to figure it out, Kirstin went all in to learn as much as possible about autoimmune, nutrition, and healing, so she closed her consulting company, took out a bunch of loans, enrolled in a holistic nutrition program, and opened the first 100% gluten-free restaurant in Arizona.

A couple years later, Anthony also enrolled in that same nutrition program and became the first Board Certified Holistic Nutritionist in Arizona. He joined Kirstin in her efforts to create a proven process to healing, not just for Kirstin, but also for others who were struggling to find their healing path.

The two have delved further into their healing passions and continue to learn as much as they can to help themselves and their clients find their most effective healing paths. In addition to his nutrition certifications, Anthony is also certified in functional lab interpretation, personal training, and took courses in biochemistry and other science- and physiology-related topics. Kirstin took her personal and professional nutrition education and added certifications in trauma healing, neurolinguistic programming, cognitive behavioral therapy, energy healing, and other emotional healing techniques.

Now, more than a decade later, Kirstin has cleared her autoimmune issues, and she and Anthony have worked with hundreds of clients to help them free themselves from their autoimmune, nagging symptoms, and related issues, too.

So, the connection between two people, which all started more than a dozen years ago with a simple email message sent through an online dating site, has resulted in hundreds of people living fuller, more optimal lives, physically, mentally, and emotionally and kicking their symptoms to the curb!

PART 1

CLARITY

What does transformational healing look like for you?

L et's get super clear on where you want to go in your health and where you are now so that we can get a better understanding of where and why you're blocked.

In this section, we're going to:

- Clarify your health goals and future vision.
- Get a clear understanding of your symptoms.
- Discuss a timeline revealing what your future holds.
- Reveal blocks that may be stopping you from reaching your health goals.

Obviously, it's up to you if you want to participate in the exercises and questions in this book. We strongly encourage you to answer all of them because they will help you uncover what is truly at the core of your symptoms and diagnosis, even if you think you already know.

They will also help you shed light on the hidden blocks stopping your healing. Things you may not be aware of because you've created defense mechanisms specifically to protect you from seeing them. The exercises and questions were designed to help you be able to open up and move beyond those defenses.

That way, the techniques, suggestions, and processes revealed to you in this book will be able to help you get on the right path to reach your personal healing.

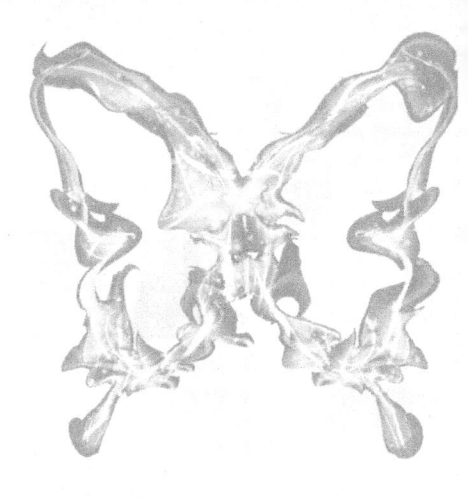

CHAPTER 1

GOALS

Breathe. Take a deep breath. Get comfortable.

When you feel stuck or have been struggling physically, mentally, or emotionally, looking for a solution, it can feel difficult to write down your goals. That's okay. It's common.

Imagine what specific things would you need to see in the next 12 weeks to know that you're on the right healing path. Write down whatever comes to mind.

Next, what would you like to see over the next 12 *months* that would indicate you were on the right path?

What are the emotional, mental, and physical indicators that would help you to know you were healing?

Think about:

- What symptoms would be in your rearview mirror?
- How would your relationships be impacted?
- What would your mornings be like?
- What impact would there be on your physical appearance?

- Would you be excelling at work or perhaps starting your own business?
- Maybe you'd like to see yourself in a completely shifted state.
- What things would you no longer be worried about?
- What would be the best part of your day?

There are no wrong answers. Write down whatever comes to mind and try not to edit yourself on what you "should" write as those answers are typically driven by feelings of guilt or shame, and don't come from your true Self. There's no "shoulding" on yourself allowed here. Write the answers that get you excited and are what you truly desire.

Jump ahead three years into the future. *What would you like to see for your life three years from now?*

If you just shut down when you read the words "three years" because you've been struggling so much that you can't even image three years from now, give yourself a moment. The answer is in there. It just may be blocked because you're afraid that you can't have what you want or that it's not possible. So, your mind is trying to protect you from that disappointment and is in fear mode.

That's common. Give yourself a minute or come back to this question after reading this story of one of our clients and what happened when she moved past her fear and was able to express her three-year goals.

Tara's Story

When we met Tara, she was 49 years old and had already undergone conventional treatment for breast cancer. The breast implants she felt pressured by her doctors to get to "help her emotional state" after her double mastectomy had triggered Lupus and psoriasis. Even though she had the implants removed, she was still struggling with severe brain fog, anxiety, depression, joint pain, exhaustion, migraines, hot flashes, acne, rashes, ringing in her ears, ovarian cysts, and a what she described as a "continual loss of words."

She had a history of mentally and emotionally abusive relationships and was living every day in basic survival mode, feeling hopeless. She had been taking medications for anxiety for nearly two decades and recalls being told from a young age that she needed to "control her feelings."

Her mental clarity had gotten so bad that doctors diagnosed her with dementia and told her that because of the speed of her decline, she should "get her affairs in order."

Tara discussed the situation with her children and partner and, as she said, "began preparing to die."

But there was a light inside of her, pushing her to keep searching for an answer. Her will to live was overriding her doctor's bleak prediction.

When we interview potential clients, we ask them to list their 12-week, 12-month, and three-year goals, just as we encouraged you to do. Often, people struggle to answer the three-year goals because they stopped being able to connect with their vision of the future. Not surprisingly, Tara was one of those people.

"I can't see that far into the future because I was told I don't have that long to live," she said. "It was hard enough coming up with the year-long goals."

"Humor me," Kirstin said. "If you were to live that long, what would you want to see for yourself three years from now?"

She thought for a moment and cautiously said, "I would want to have a career, one that would help people like me who were suffering and wanted answers."

During the program, clients regularly meet with a Nourish Coach one-on-one to review their goals and check in to see they are on track. In addition to her long-term goal of having a career helping others, Tara also wanted to:

- Have more energy.
- Understand what her body needed and didn't need.
- Reduce or eliminate symptoms.
- Regain her self-worth and balance.

- Find purpose in her life.
- Learn to relax.
- Have social energy.
- Eliminate feelings of hopelessness.
- No longer be dependent on medication.

Though she was nervous, Tara jumped into the program with both feet. She followed her personal meal plan and fitness recommendations, and she studied the learning modules. Most importantly, she attended the coaching clinics and one-on-one coaching appointments. She asked questions, saw reflections of herself through the healing journeys of others, and allowed herself to be vulnerable. She approached the exercises and homework suggested to her with curiosity and openness.

Within six months, symptoms such as psoriasis, acne, rashes, hot flashes, and migraines were completely gone, and challenges such as hopelessness, fear, depression, anxiety, joint pain, and tinnitus had moved from an 8 or 9 (10 being the most severe) to a 2!

The most wonderful of all of her accomplishments was that by the six-month mark, Tara was already in school learning a specific form of hypnosis and planning her career as a healer! So, she was well on her way to hitting her three-year goals, in only a few months!

By her year anniversary, Tara had essentially eliminated nearly all of her symptoms. She allowed herself to admit that though she always dreamed of living by the beach, that after living in a beach house for the past several years, she realized that she really only loves beach houses on vacation. So, she sold her "dream house" and moved to one that better supported her soul so she can continue to thrive, heal, and get even closer to her true Self and her core purpose, and live out her true dream of transforming her health.

Tara would absolutely tell you that she is grateful every day for her healing journey and the success that she's had. But she would also tell you that it wasn't necessarily easy. She was rewarded, like hundreds of other clients we've had the privilege of working with, because she believed in the voice telling her to trust and move toward healing. She showed up for herself emotionally, mentally, and physically by making herself a priority and taking advantage of the tools and support available to her.

And, like Meghan's story, and other stories you'll come across in this book, Tara's story is wonderful, but her success isn't a miracle. It's what happens when you listen to the conversation from your body, and give it what it's asking for to heal.

And that kind of healing is available to *anyone* who is open to putting themselves first, accepting the right support, and doing the work!

Remember, this exercise is to help you open up and really see what is possible in the future, which you need to trigger transformational healing.

Chapter Takeaways

- What are the top five things would you like to happen in the next three months, 12 months, and three years that would indicate you were on the right healing path?

- True healing requires openness, curiosity, and willingness to making changes in your life.

- Everyone has the inherit ability to heal and get on the right path.

- When you put yourself first, it has a profound impact on your healing trajectory

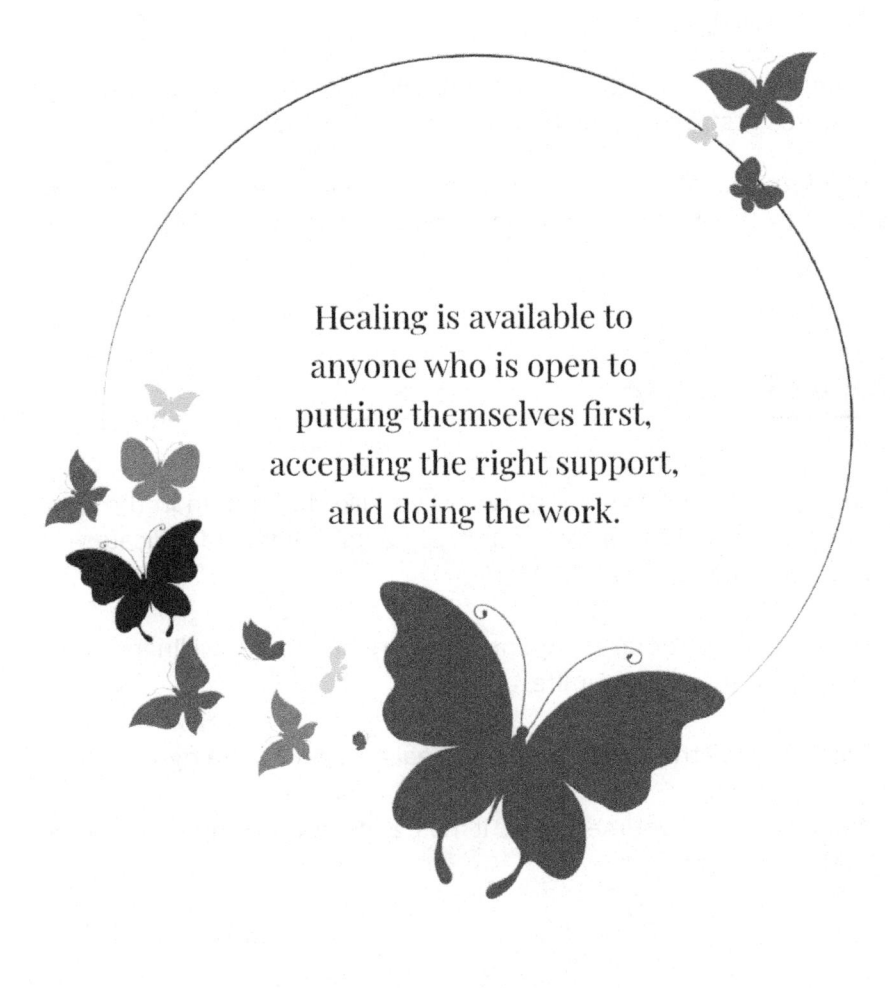

Healing is available to anyone who is open to putting themselves first, accepting the right support, and doing the work.

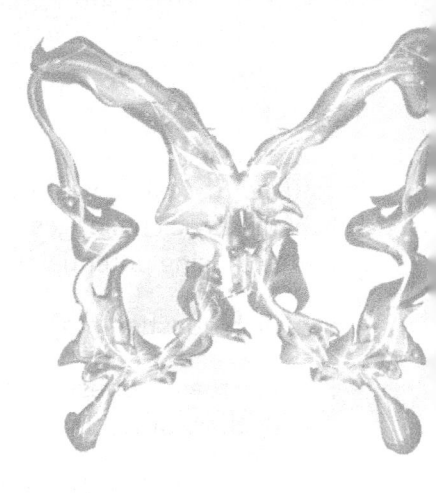

CHAPTER 2

SYMPTOMS

Now that you've taken a peek into your future and listed your true core desires, list all of your symptoms. Include anything in your life right now that feels out of balance physically, mentally, or emotionally.

Here are some questions to help you create your own list:

- What are my current symptoms?
- What does my sleep look like?
- What are my bowels doing?
- What is going on with my thoughts?
- What's going on in my relationships?
- What's my relationship to food?
- How do I feel about myself?
- How do I feel about the world around me?
- What things keep popping up that feel out of balance that don't feel right or good?

The answers to these questions will help you flesh out symptoms and messages from your body which you may have overlooked or become so used to dealing with that you no longer even notice them. Shining light on these challenges will give you insight into blocks or underlying issues causing potential havoc in your body.

This next question may be difficult, but it's important.

If I were really honest with myself, how long have I been experiencing signals that something just wasn't right?

Understanding where you first started feeling out of balance and really started noticing signs of inflammation is helpful to see some of the more subtle ways your body was trying to communicate with you. This awareness, as we will discuss in more detail throughout the book, will help you in your healing process.

Example

The symptoms Kirstin experienced alerting her to the eventual diagnosis of celiac disease and Hashimoto's started way before the doctors diagnosed her in her 30s. There were many signs that began decades before.

- The "seasonal allergies" she had for as long as she could remember.
- The intense shoulder tightness her gymnastics and softball coaches commented about often.
- Swollen tonsils, eustachian tube inflammation, sinus infections.... throughout childhood and into adulthood.
- Stomach aches, nausea, and digestive issues as a preteen and into adulthood.
- Irregular periods, dizziness, severe cramping, hormonal migraines, and bloating associated with her cycle. Heavy pain killers and birth control were prescribed, which created their own set of symptoms.
- Intense mood swings including anger, depression, rage, panic attacks, and sadness that she suppressed most of the time.
- Embarrassing and painful cystic acne that started in early adulthood.

- Urinary tract infections, yeast infections, and unexplained blood in the urine, which put her on a path of visits with specialists and many invasive and painful testing that never produced any insight.
- Weight gain that began in early adulthood and wouldn't budge even with extreme cardio, special diets, and personal training.
- The "random" severe allergic reactions that would happen causing any combination of hives, swelling, shortness of breath, and other immune responses.
- Shingles multiple times.

There were many more, but you probably get the idea.

The point is: her body was communicating to let her know it was out of balance, just as yours is right now. Have you noticed? Have you been listening? How long has it been trying to get your attention?

List out all of the symptoms, signs, and messages your body has been sending you, trying to alert you to the fact that it was in trouble.

Symptoms: Impact

Next, list the impact that those symptoms have been having on your life.

- Are you canceling appointments with people or not even bothering to make plans with friends anymore because you just don't want to cancel?
- What are you unable to do physically?
- Have you stopped getting down on the floor to play with your children or grandchildren because you're in pain?
- What are you not able to do because of your symptoms?
- What excuses or stories do you tell people to avoid explaining what you're going through?
- How much time do you spend preplanning all of your food because

it seems like everything you eat makes you sick?

- Rather than enjoying your vacations, do you find yourself hyper-focused on where the bathrooms are at all times because you have IBS/IBD or Crohn's disease and you are concerned that, at any moment, you could have an accident?

How are my symptoms impacting my goals?

List all the ways your symptoms are stopping, influencing, or impeding your goals in life. Did you think you were going to be farther along by now, but symptoms are slowing your down? Have you given up on any dreams because you can no longer focus on anything but your fatigue, pain, or frustration? Get real about what's going on and bring your current experience out into the open. When you stop dismissing or trying to hide from the truth is when you can finally move onto your unique healing path.

Chapter Takeaways

- When you are honest with yourself and get clear on what symptoms you are experiencing and how long they've been impacting your life, it's easier to understand the conversation your body has been trying to have with you.

- It's easy to minimize symptoms and brush them off by ignoring them, suppressing them with medication, or justifying them by blaming age, circumstance, or "stress." Addressing them directly is the only way to try get a solution.

- Symptoms are the body's way of communicating with you. Are you listening?

CHAPTER 3

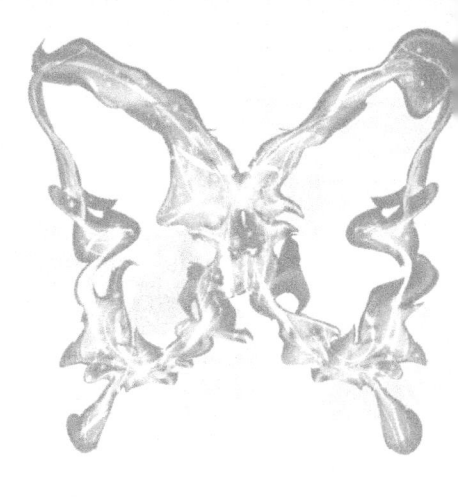

TIMELINE

The question everyone wants to know is: once I find the right healing path, how long will it take me to heal?

This is an important question. So, let's discuss what impacts the healing trajectory by using the following timeline model.

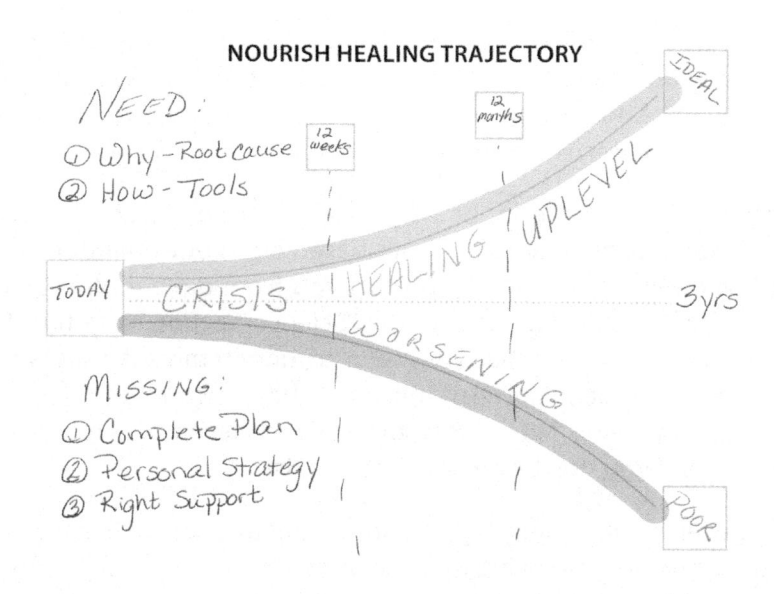

NOURISH HEALING TRAJECTORY

NEED:
① Why - Root Cause
② How - Tools

TODAY — CRISIS — 12 weeks — HEALING — 12 months — UPLEVEL — IDEAL

WORSENING — 3yrs — POOR

MISSING:
① Complete Plan
② Personal Strategy
③ Right Support

The Nourish Healing Trajectory model shows two different health trajectories over the course of three years, with marks at 12 weeks and at 12 months. The top trajectory is ideal. The bottom one is a poor health trajectory.

The starting point is at the left side of the model. Imagine you are at that starting point right now. If nothing changes, what do you imagine your health will look like in three years? Which health trajectory do you think you'll be on? Ideal or poor? How will this impact your daily life? How will this impact your future plans? How will this impact your goals, relationships, and life purpose?

Now, let's compare this to a different outcome. Imagine that you are right now at the starting point on the left, but you **have what you need to heal** and you take action and begin making those changes today. Imagine what your health will look like in three years. What impact will that have on your goals, experiences, relationships, and life?

Over time, the difference between the poor health trajectory and the ideal health trajectory will become more obvious and further apart. So the sooner you get started and take action, the sooner you can experience your ideal healthy life!

Since we are hard-wired to do what our subconscious perceives is safe, we typically do, think, and behave in ways we think will keep us out of danger. One of the ways the subconscious determines what is safe is based on the patterns we participate in and are familiar with.

Whatever state you are in: healthy, sick, frustrated, scared, anxious, excited, worried, or symptomatic, it's based on a series of patterns the body has determined will help protect you from danger. We will dive deeper into this concept later in the "Science Section" and the "Soul Section," but for now, what you need to understand is that we are hard-wired to repeat patterns because the subconscious connects patterns with being safe. Most of these patterns are running on autopilot, and you don't even know they exist.

So whatever health trajectory you are on (ideal or poor), it's primarily because of these underlying familiar patterns.

Even though the pattern that feels familiar might be anxiety, if your body is familiar with it and thinks the anxiety is keeping you safe, then not only will it resist changing that pattern, it might even associate the feeling of calm with danger because calm is not your familiar pattern.

Seems backwards, right?

We weren't wired for happiness or even for good health. We were wired to stay safe. So, if your subconscious is familiar with feeling anxious, then it will continue to perpetuate the anxiety because it thinks the anxiety is helping you stay safe.

If it's unfamiliar with feeling calm, then calm may actually trigger you into feeling unsafe.

Familiar equals safe. Unfamiliar equals danger.

Your system is constantly projecting a movie of what your life will be like in the future, based on familiar patterns from the past. So, it already sees your trajectory 12 weeks out, 12 months out, and three years out. And the decisions you make today are based on this future projection.

Your subconscious brain is constantly looking for evidence that you are on the right path to get you to the "safest" point. And for many, the safest point is actually on the poor health trajectory, **because it feels familiar.**

If you have been participating in patterns that create poor health, but those patterns are connected to your version of safety or comfort, then you will stay on the poor health trajectory.

For example, imagine that when you were a child, whenever something "bad" happened to you, your mother gave you candy to "cheer you up." You may have connected the candy to feeling good, and safe, and comforted. Therefore, any time you feel "bad" emotionally, mentally, or physically, your brain jumps to the safe pattern of eating candy to feel better.

Without realizing it, you find yourself reaching for sweets at any sign of "danger," even when you're not hungry. When you were told that you labs results showed signs of diabetes, you actually found yourself eating more sweets to offset the fear you have of getting sick like your grandmother who eventually died of complications of diabetes.

Logically, you know eating sweets isn't a healthy choice and leads to poor health, but your subconscious still drives you to eating those sweets to keep you "safe."

The good news is that you can rewire these familiar patterns and flip yourself to the ideal health trajectory. You are not locked forever on the poor health trajectory.

We will cover in more detail what you need in order to rewire your system throughout the remainder of this book.

First, let's get super real about your trajectory by taking a moment to answer the question below with radical honesty.

If my current life trajectory does not change, what will my life look like in three years?

The reason it's critical to your healing to answer this question as honestly as possible, and to spend quality time answering all the questions and exercises in this book, is because your subconscious is currently watching its version of your life trajectory, based on your interpretation of what's happened to you so far.

And that vision is playing like a movie beneath the surface without you even realizing it, driving your beliefs, decisions, and actions all day long. So, unless you get real and bring this underlying vision to the surface and truly see it, then you cannot begin to rewire it. You have to know what you are rewiring to do it successfully.

When we first meet clients, they are in what we would call the "crisis state." What they really want to be in is a "healing state." You cannot be in crisis and healing simultaneously. If you are in crisis, your body sends all its resources to handle the crisis, leaving no resources available for healing.

For example, banging your head against the wall until you get a headache causes a crisis situation. Just because you take a pain killer and suppress the pain doesn't mean you are healed. It only means you have covered up the signal the body is using to alert you to the crisis.

Once the medication wears off, if you are still causing crisis by banging your head, not only will the headache return but also you most likely have caused more damage in the process.

The problem is that *the cause of the crisis* (the banging of the head) wasn't resolved. And if the cause isn't discovered and resolved, even if the pain has subsided temporarily, the damage will continue, and healing cannot happen.

Looking back at the timeline model, what we've found is that it takes most people about 12 weeks to move out of the crisis stage and into the healing stage, with the right tools and support.

In order to move into healing, you need two important pieces:

1. Uncovering physical, mental, and emotional root causes to *why* you are on the poor health trajectory.
2. *How* to use the tools you need to dissolve those issues.

This doesn't mean that in 12 weeks you will always know every reason why you're in crisis and all of the tools to help dissolve those issues. Not every cause is ready to surface right away. Most people need to build some emotional and physical strength, as well as skills to locate and manage the discoveries when they do surface. True self-discovery is a life long journey.

However, 12 weeks is a solid amount of time to shed light on, and surface some of the most destructive root causes hiding in the shadows causing some of the most challenging of symptoms, and to really begin seeing a shift in those symptoms. Once you surface these blocks and learn how to use the best tools for your specific situation, you then have to learn how to use those tools effectively and consistently so as not to slide back into old patterns of false safety. It's at this point that clients feel like they're really coming out of the fog and feeling like themselves again. From there most people need about three to 12 months to then lock in the new patterns and give the body time to heal from the damage that may have been going on for 20 or 40 years.

After about a year, that's when people hit a whole new level of healing, fulfillment, and joy. At this stage, clients are no longer hyper focused on eliminating symptoms and trying to function at a "normal level." They are upleveling their systems and not just "getting their lives back"; they are often living their dream lives. They are traveling, starting businesses, growing their families, getting advanced degrees, and training for fitness competitions. They are not just participating in life; they are living fully, expressing themselves wholly, and unapologetically dancing in their truest selves.

Once you move out of crisis and into true healing, only then can you experience who you really are and move toward your dream life. The energy shift to transformational healing is amazing and one that everyone can experience once they know how.

Chapter Takeaways

- Your healing trajectory is largely influenced by the patterns you repeat at a subconscious level to stay "safe," which you usually aren't even aware is happening.

- Understanding what is impacting your healing trajectory, and the underlying physical, mental, and emotional root causes of symptoms is crucial to finding the right healing path.

- Once you understand what's at the root of symptoms and disease, you need the right tools and support to be able to shift off the poor health trajectory, and create new patterns that feel safe.

CHAPTER 4

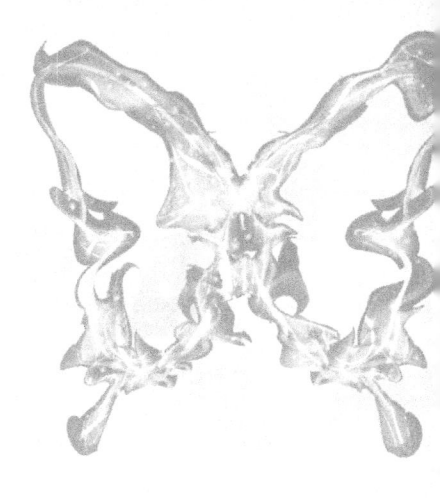

TRIGGERS, TRAUMAS, AND BLOCKS

When dealing with autoimmune, illness, cancer, and other inflammatory health problems, there are three prongs that converge to create the disease.

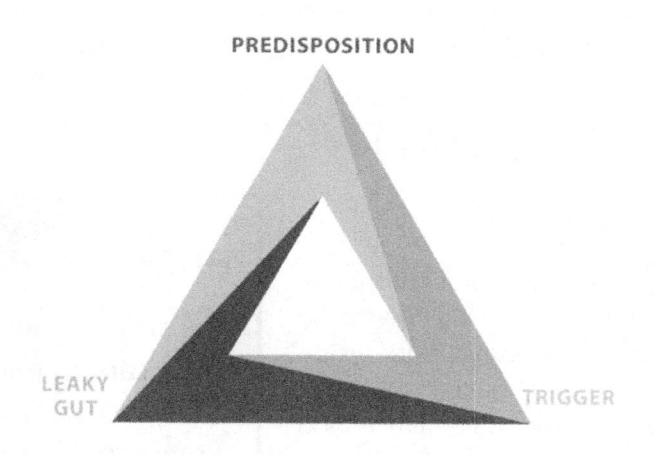

- **Predisposition.** This means there is a genetic component to the illness or disease. This doesn't mean that because one of your parents had an autoimmune condition that you automatically have autoimmune disease. It means that you are *predisposed* to autoimmune problems, but the expression of those genes depends upon the influence of environment. We will get into much more depth on this issue when discussing epigenetics in Chapter 18 in the "Science Section".

- **Leaky Gut.** Again, this will be covered in more depth in Chapter 9: Food in the "Nutrition Section" of the book, but essentially, this means the lining of the gut was weakened by physical, emotional, and/or environmental toxins. This weakening, allowed food particles to permeate through the gut lining into the blood system, causing inflammation, food sensitivities, low nutrient absorption, and other problems, putting the body on high alert and triggering various fight-or-flight responses.

- **Triggers.** A trigger is a cause or combination of causes that tip the body over into a state of danger, inflammation, or disease and pushes the system into a state of ill health. A trigger can be any emotional, mental, physical, or environmental cause that the body perceives as traumatic. Examples of common triggers are pregnancy, abuse, or mold exposure. We will be exploring multiple different types of triggers throughout the rest of this book, but right now, let's delve a little bit more into some of the emotional ones.

Understanding Emotional Triggers

Ninety percent of your thoughts, beliefs, and actions are driven by your subconscious brain. Your vision of the future is based on your perception of the past. Once you understand that, you can then begin to understand why you're stuck in patterns keeping you tied to a poor health trajectory and why you may not even realize there is another trajectory available to you.

> **HACK:**
>
> The subconscious brain cannot tell the difference between a memory, a dream, a current experience, and a future vision. The conscious brain sorts all of that out.

Chapter 4 - Triggers, Traumas, and Blocks

If the conscious brain is the only part that can recognize the difference between your thoughts, imagination, and memories, but your subconscious is driving 90% of your thoughts, beliefs, and actions, then this means your subconscious is controlling your ability to heal.

That's a big deal.

To get the healing results you want, especially if you find yourself getting worse over time, you have to know how to hack into those hidden patterns and beliefs hiding in your subconscious.

When has any practitioner ever included that in your healing plan?

If that hasn't been an integral part of your journey so far, that's most likely a big reason (if not the biggest reason) you are currently struggling right now.

Let's check in. What are you feeling right now?

Are you excited because you finally see an opening at the end of the tunnel?

Are you perhaps getting anxious because you are wondering if it's too late for you and that perhaps you are too sick to stop the train and change directions?

Is a little (or maybe not so little) voice saying:

- What if I can't have my vision of a healthy life?
- What if I'm too sick to heal?
- What if I'm incapable of making the changes necessary?
- What if I do all of the work, and healing just isn't available to me?

If you're blocking the vision of your healed self out of fear, then it is critical you learn how to dissolve that fear and allow yourself to see a future vision of the healed you.

The good news is: The answer on how to do that is in this book.

So, take a deep breath. Realize that the fear is simply an *old pattern* based on your *perception* of past experiences. *It doesn't mean the fear is true.* It's just the hardwiring in your subconscious trying to keep you safe.

And that wiring, can be rewired. We do it with our clients every day. And you can do it, too.

You're in the right place. Keep reading.

We're going to dig deeper and reveal what you need to shine light into the subconscious paradigm so you can see what's holding you back, and move from the poor health trajectory to your ideal trajectory.

Chapter Takeaways

- Disease, especially autoimmune, is typically caused by a combination of three issues: genetic predisposition, leaky gut, and emotional, physical, and/or environmental "triggers."

- Your subconscious drives 90% of your thoughts, beliefs, and actions. Which means it is largely in control of your ability to heal.

- Surfacing and dissolving hidden negative patterns of belief must be addressed in order to find long-term, whole healing.

CHAPTER 5

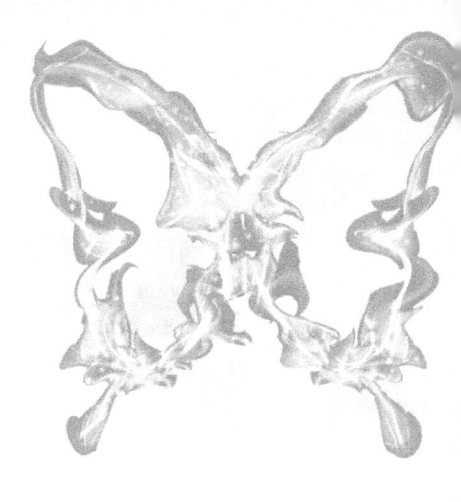

SELF ATTACK

Statistically, if you've been diagnosed with one autoimmune disease, there's another one coming down the pike. **The immune system attacking you is the problem,** though the conventional medical community puts the focus on the part of the body **being attacked.**

When you have Hashimoto's for example, your thyroid isn't the problem; your immune system attacking your thyroid: that's the problem. If you take medication to force the thyroid to "behave properly" then you are at best, suppressing symptoms temporarily. If you don't address the cause (the thyroid being attacked by the immune system), then you are still in trouble and the crisis is still happening.

Why would your immune system, which is designed to protect you and help you heal, attack you?

It's not because it's "overactive" as you've probably been told. It's because the immune system is doing its job of trying to protect you, but it's *confused*.

When you are out of alignment with who you truly are, this creates imbalance and confusion within your system. When your body is attacking you, it's a sign that it doesn't recognize what it's attacking is part of you.

It thinks what it's attacking is a *threat* to you.

When you suppress who you truly are through medication, have a low sense of self worth, or try to be something other than who you really are, this creates *confusion.*

Suppression of self-expression will set off internal alarms creating conflict and ultimately, if not addressed, it will lead to a self-attack in an effort to set you free.

So, if you suppress your true Self, it can create confusion and fear and trigger an attack.

If you constantly berate yourself and think you're not good enough, it can create confusion that you are the enemy and trigger an attack. If you consume harmful foods, use toxic products, or participate in dangerous activities, the only way to get your attention and "protect you" from these choices might be through self-attack.

When we behave out of alignment with our true Self is when you will see symptoms, illness, and disease. It's the body's internal defense system trying to keep us from harm, which ironically triggers an attack on Self.

It's the literal meaning to the commonly paraphrased quote by philosopher Friedrich Nietzche: We are our own worst enemy.

Chapter Takeaways

- Autoimmune disease is your immune system attacking a part of you. Treating the part of the body being attacked doesn't correct the root issue causing the attack. The focus must be placed on stopping the immune system from attacking what it's supposed to be protecting.

- Addressing and dissolving negative patterns and beliefs is part of the healing process.

- Being out of alignment with who you are at your core creates imbalance and confusion. Autoimmune disease is an indication that the body doesn't recognize you and you are not being true to Self.

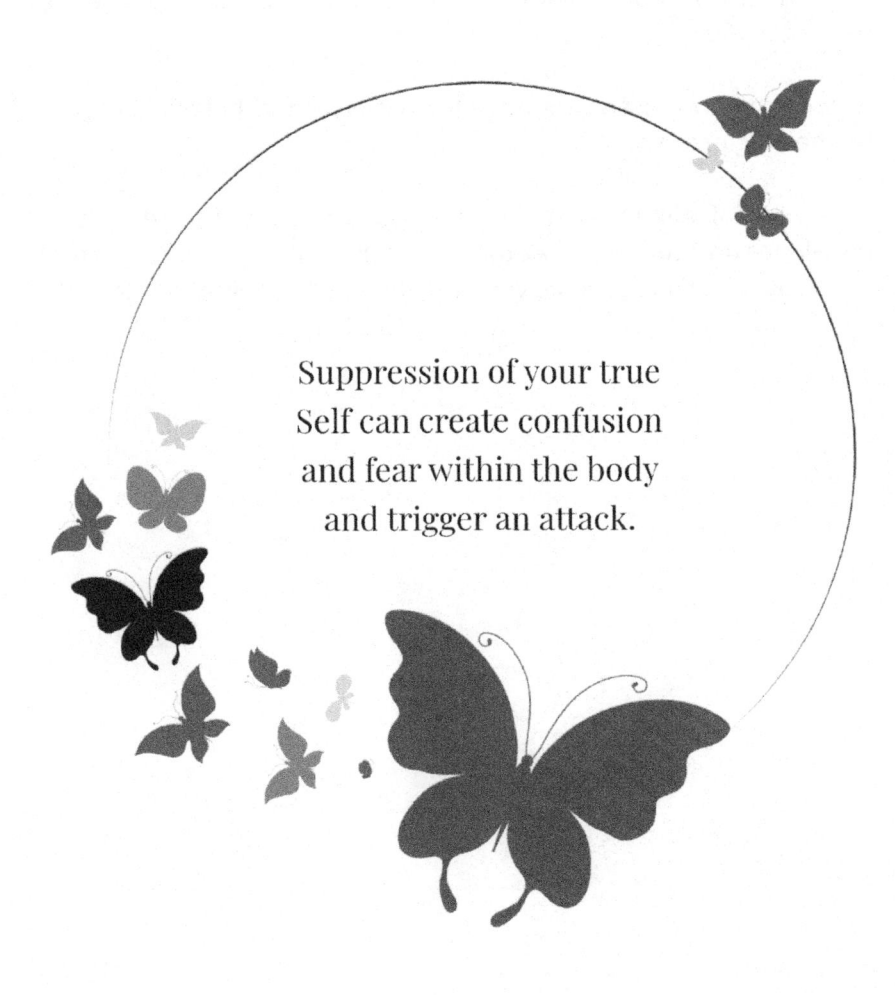

Suppression of your true
Self can create confusion
and fear within the body
and trigger an attack.

CHAPTER 6

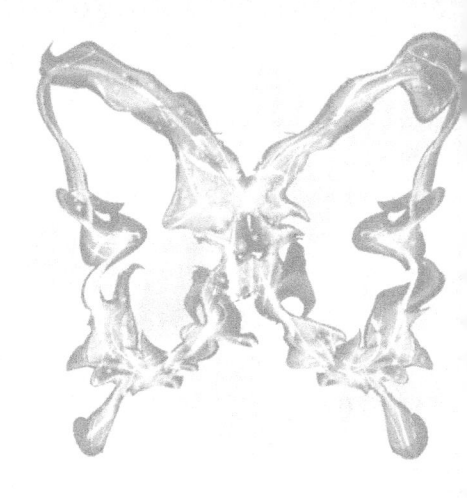

HIDDEN DRIVERS

In order for you to get optimal results from the exercises in this book and understand why your body isn't feeling balanced, you need to understand what's driving you subconsciously. The questions and the exercises will help you start cracking open hidden messages, conversations, and drivers going on beneath the surface.

Lori's Story

Before we get any deeper, here's an example of a hidden driver we helped a client uncover that was at the core of her most frustrating symptom.

Lori had been working with us for several months and she was doing well stopping symptoms and beginning to heal. She attended one of Kirstin's client coaching clinics and said: "I'm so frustrated. I'm doing so well with all my other symptoms, but I don't know why I'm still not losing weight."

Kirstin replied: "Sounds like your subconscious believes that it's safer for you to hold onto the weight than to release it."

Lori: "Well, that sounds ridiculous. Why would my body think it was safer to be fat?"

Kirstin: "The subconscious is not wired for happiness, health, or logic. It's wired to keep us safe. Which means, whatever is happening in our system, it's because, at the subconscious level, we feel it is keeping us safe."

Lori still didn't like that, but she was open and willing to do what she had to do to change her subconscious belief.

Kirstin assigned an exercise to list 30 reasons her body might feel safer by holding onto the excess weight.

A week later, she presented a list of only 11 reasons, but the fourth one revealed her block.

Her answer to number four was "I won't starve" and she had written "Haha!" next to it.

Kirstin locked right into Lori's answer for number four and said to her: "Tell me about a time when you were starving," and Lori's entire body shifted. The expression on her face got more serious and you could tell that a nerve had been hit.

More than 40 years ago, when Lori was only 22, her abusive husband left her and their two babies to fend for themselves. She dug deep and found the courage to go back to school while holding down multiple jobs to cover the bills. As she explained, there were many nights the kids got fed, but she didn't.

Though she's now an electrical engineer, has a stable job,

> **HACK:**
> Many people use humor to protect themselves from dealing with underlying blocks. The humor is often a big arrow pointing to a core issue creating imbalance in the body and a message from the subconscious that we're missing something. So, pay closer attention when and where you use humor or sarcasm. There may be a gem hidden right below the surface.

lives in a safe area, and her kids are long grown with their own children, her body was still anchored to that trauma.

Her subconscious paradigm still believed that at any moment, she could be in a situation where she may starve. This underlying belief was driving hidden thoughts and caused her to take action to protect herself from that ever-lurking danger.

For example, even though Lori lived alone, she had an extra freezer heavily stocked with food. The message running on autopilot in her subconscious repeating, "You could starve at any moment," sent signals to her body to slow down metabolism and hold onto excess weight to protect her from the danger.

And because it happened so many years ago, it never occurred to her that it was still a very real belief today.

Now that it surfaced, she could see the direct connection to the trauma and how it was driving her current thoughts and behavior. She was able to use the additional tools we gave her to process it and release the fear anchored to it.

Just a few days after surfacing this block, Lori began to lose weight. We continued to work on pulling threads attached to this specific trauma and helping Lori feel more connected, balanced, and loved.

Chapter Takeaways

- The subconscious isn't wired for happiness, health, or logic. It's wired to keep us safe. So, it sticks with what is familiar and typically rejects new behaviors, thoughts, or actions.

- Symptoms reveal information when you know how and where to look. Every symptom means something. It's a communication from your body giving you clues to why your body is behaving the way it is.

- What is your most stubborn symptom? It's most likely the key to a treasure chest of healing information.

CHAPTER 7

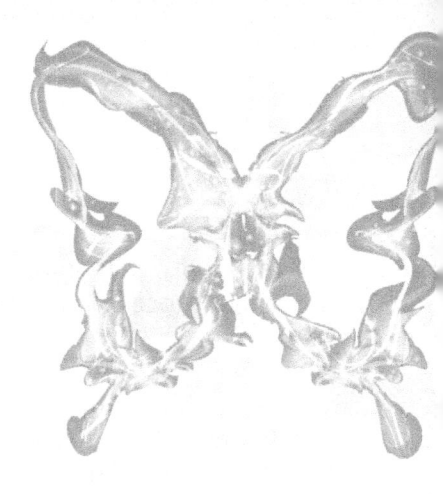

WHAT IS (NEGATIVE) TRAUMA?

So often, people don't understand what their body considers trauma; therefore, they don't even know what they're looking to uncover.

Trauma is a shocking moment which challenged your paradigm or reinforced it, creating a deep physical, mental, and emotional connection to that experience. A negative trauma is a shocking moment your body decided was a threat to your survival based on its perception of that moment filtered through past experiences and emotional responses. Later in Chapter 23: Understanding Trauma, we will discuss both negative trauma and the often-overlooked concept of positive trauma. For right now, we're going to look at a more traditional view of how (negative) trauma impacts the body.

Perceived danger puts the body on high alert, and it looks for evidence that the threat is real and how threatening the danger is. If the perceived danger is high, physical, mental, and emotional connections experienced in that moment get locked into the system to prepare you to run or fight that danger in case something similar should happen again.

In Lori's case, her body was holding on to extra weight as a defense mechanism against starving. It essentially bubble-wrapped her with fat to protect her from the danger that was still very real in her subconscious mind.

It was also causing her body to stay in fight-or-flight mode, which was keeping other processes suppressed like digestion, hormone balance, and the ability to manage inflammation. We will get into more detail about that process later in this book.

What we want to focus on now is how an experience from the past, no matter how long ago it happened, can still drive thoughts, feelings, beliefs, and actions right now. Because the subconscious brain doesn't function from the idea of linear time like the conscious brain does.

As far as the subconscious is concerned, everything connected to a perceived trauma (emotions, feelings, thoughts, and even sensations like temperature, sounds, and smells) is being triggered and it feels like it's happening in real time. Let's dig deeper into what that means.

Moments that happened 40 years ago, can still trigger a response from the body as if it were happening *in this moment*. And the danger can feel just as real now as it did four decades ago. Even though Lori was well out of danger of starving, her subconscious was sending out a distress signal that, at any minute, she may not have access to enough food. So, she kept her extra freezer stocked full of food, she always finished everything on her plate even after she was full, and her body held onto extra weight to protect her from the danger of starving. Until Lori addressed this hidden belief, the danger was very real, and it wasn't just a memory of the past; her subconscious believed it was still a current and present threat.

Here's what this means for you: if you have a symptom that is still hanging around even though you feel like you've "tried everything" but it just refuses to go away, then it is likely something is lodged in your subconscious, causing your body to think that it is safer to have that symptom than not to have it.

It could be a belief that unless you put everyone else's needs before your own, you are "selfish." Because when you grew up, your mother often told you to "Stop being so selfish!"

Or it may be because you were praised for how much of a "little helper" you were, caring for your younger brothers and sisters when you mom was sick.

Or it may be because your father didn't notice you until you brought him a beer or helped him clean up his workbench in the garage. So, you learned early to pay attention to his needs before your own.

A seemingly innocent message anchored at an early age can drive behavior well into adulthood.

This is why so many people, especially mothers and caregivers, often put themselves at the bottom of the list of priorities and then end up becoming sick. How can you give 100% of yourself if you are not feeling 100%?

The underlying message that your survival depends on caring for others first can get anchored into the paradigm and run on autopilot on a constant loop. Even when you know you need to focus on yourself first, without some specific rewiring of that underlying message, you will keep putting everyone else first at the detriment of your own health.

Chapter Takeaways

- Trauma is something your body believed was a threat to your survival based on your perception of the experience at that moment.

- The subconscious brain cannot determine the difference between a past memory, a future vision, or a current experience. It balls them all up together, causing or retriggering physical, emotional, and mental reactions in real time.

- Lingering symptoms mean your body feels safer holding onto the symptom than releasing it. That specific symptom is connected to a specific moment, typically compounded by many additional moments over time, that your subconscious has connected to being "safe." When you understand where that moment originated, you will be able to create a plan on how to dismantle the connection that symptom has to feeling safe.

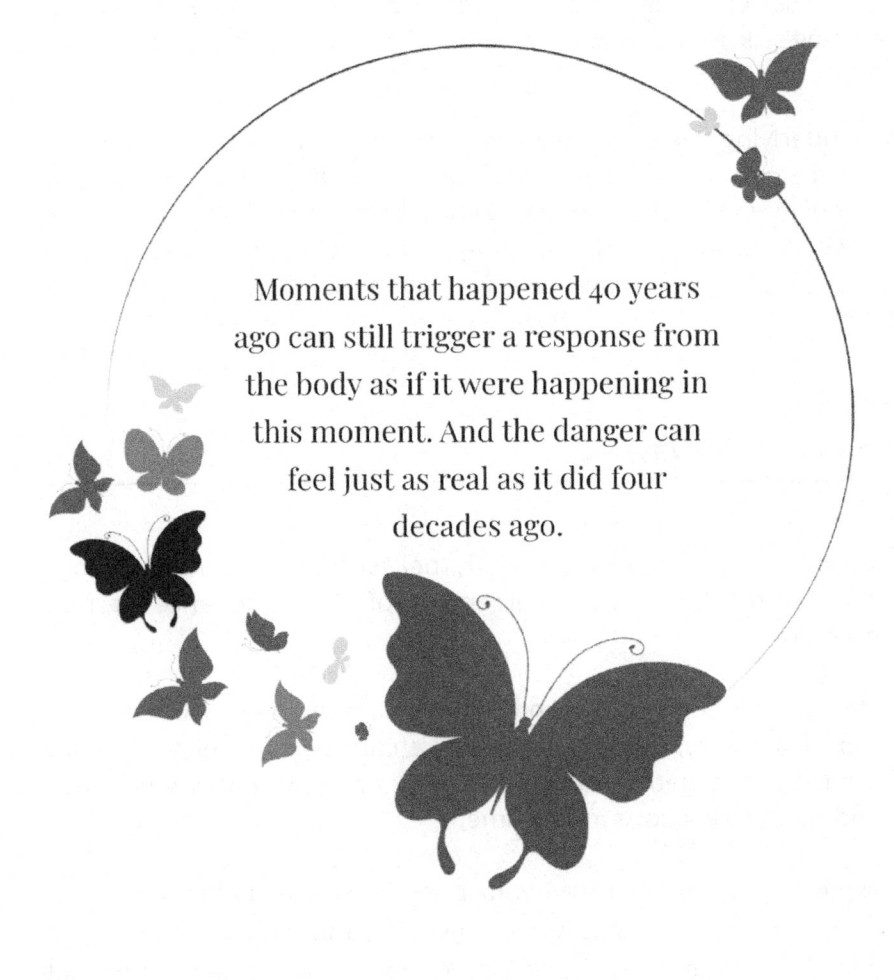

Moments that happened 40 years ago can still trigger a response from the body as if it were happening in this moment. And the danger can feel just as real as it did four decades ago.

CHAPTER 8

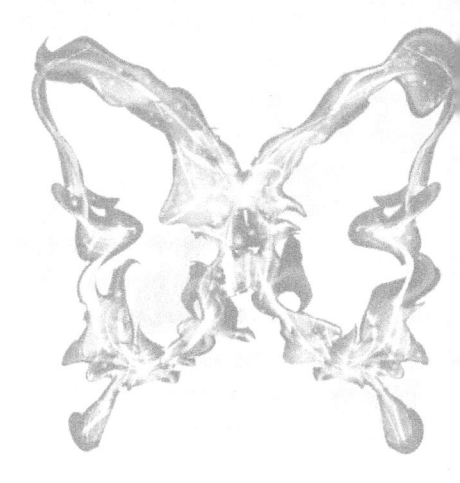

BLOCKS ARE THERE TO KEEP YOU SAFE

Hundreds of thoughts, behaviors, and actions are being controlled by your underlying connection to what is safe, and many of them are the reason you are stuck.

Maybe you are eating lots of sugar or processed foods. You may even crave those things and feel driven to eat them. That's a direct message from your subconscious that eating something sweet or processed will make you feel safe, even if it's just momentary. Then you get stuck in a cycle when you feel better in the moment as "feel good" chemicals are released in the body, and you feel comforted. This then leads to addictions to the emotions and memories connected to eating the sweets, the "feel good" chemicals impacting the body, and the avoidance of the underlying core problem.

Perhaps rather than trying to feel good, you are doing the opposite and trying to suppress bad feelings by participating in mind-numbing activities like hours of TV, Candy Crush, and social media. Or you're leaning on alcohol, medication, overeating, recreational drugs, or other substance to help you avoid feeling what you're feeling. Even seemingly healthy activities such as working out can be used to ignore underlying blocks. People use them to convince themselves that "everything is fine." We often have clients who were using working out as a way to avoid what they are actually feeling and what their body was trying to communicate.

If you find yourself hyper-focused on controlling every single thing around you like how the dishes are loaded into the dishwasher, the choices that your daughter is making for her wedding, or micromanaging your staff, this is typically a sign that there's an underlying driver making you feel out of control, overwhelmed, or scared.

These are all messages, telling you there's something hiding in the shadows of your subconscious, driving your actions, and influencing the results that you're getting.

This isn't your conscious or "intellectual thinking" brain. This is the subconscious "animal brain" delivering the message that changing is more dangerous than continuing the current pattern. It's what's keeping you on the poor health trajectory and blocking you from moving (or even seeing) your ideal health trajectory.

When you understand the power of your subconscious mind and become more aware of the underlying drivers that are truly important to you, this will bring your consciousness into the conversation, which is the only way to change your trajectory.

> **HACK:**
>
> The questions posed at the beginning of this book are a way to hack right into your subconscious mind and shed light on your underlying fears and belief blocks directly tied to your healing trajectory.

If you raised your hand high at the beginning of this book and, when asked if you wanted transformational healing, you said, "Me, me, me! I do! I do!" then you'll spend time answering these questions in depth.

Take time to truly imagine your ideal health trajectory at 12 weeks, 12 months, and three years.

Get honest and clear about your symptoms, when they really started, and how they are impacting every aspect of your life.

What are they stopping you from doing or causing you to have to do that you don't enjoy?

How are they impacting the people around you?

Are you okay with what happens in the next three years if nothing changes and your health trajectory continues down the path it's on?

When answering these questions, check in with yourself and how you feel physically, mentally, and emotionally. This will give you insight into where some of the hidden blocks are.

If you find yourself wanting to skip the questions because they're "not important" or because it hurts too much to answer them, then it's an even bigger indicator that they are exactly the questions you need to answer.

We promised we were going to help show you how to get the answers you're looking for. And this is one of the ways to do it.

Chapter Takeaways

- The subconscious is constantly on the lookout to determine what is safe and what is dangerous. All your thoughts, behaviors, and actions are being driven by what your subconscious connects to safety.

- Getting clear with what your symptoms are stopping you from doing, what they are preventing you from enjoying, and how they are impacting your life and the people around you will help you connect more deeply with how seriously your body is trying to get your attention and where to locate some hidden blocks causing your current life experience.

- When you stop and truly listen to your body, and really hear what it's trying to tell you, it will open up a treasure chest of details, which will lead you to healing.

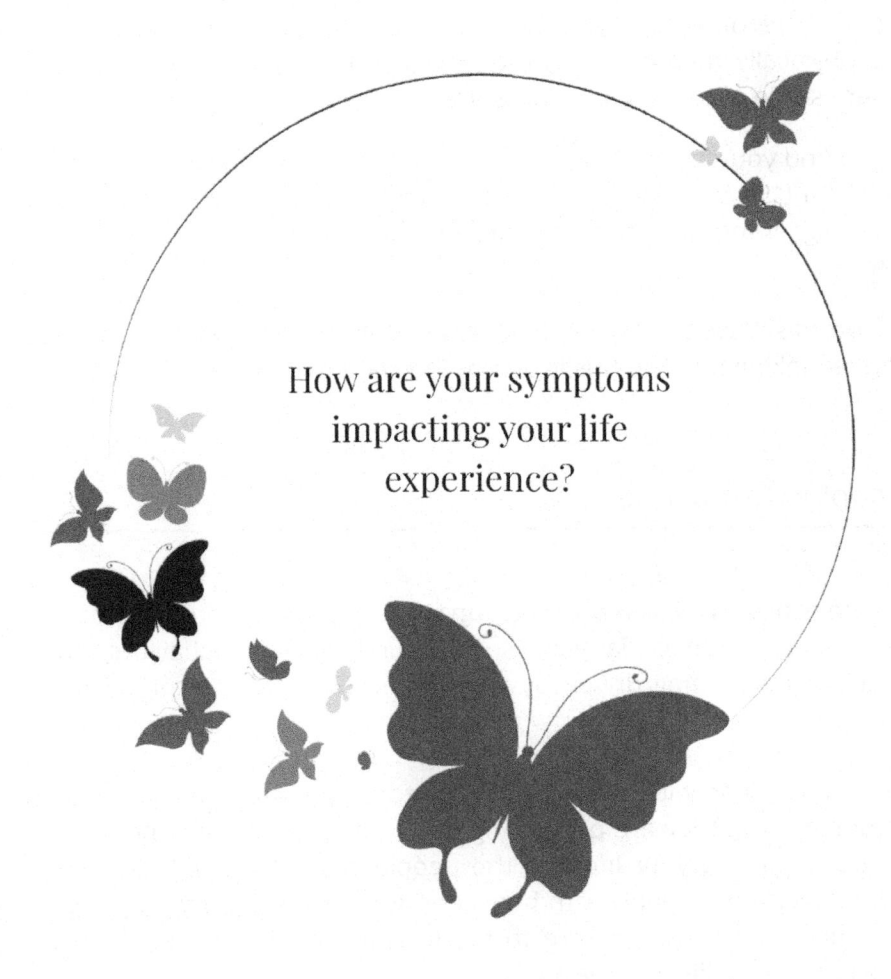

How are your symptoms impacting your life experience?

PART 2

NUTRITION

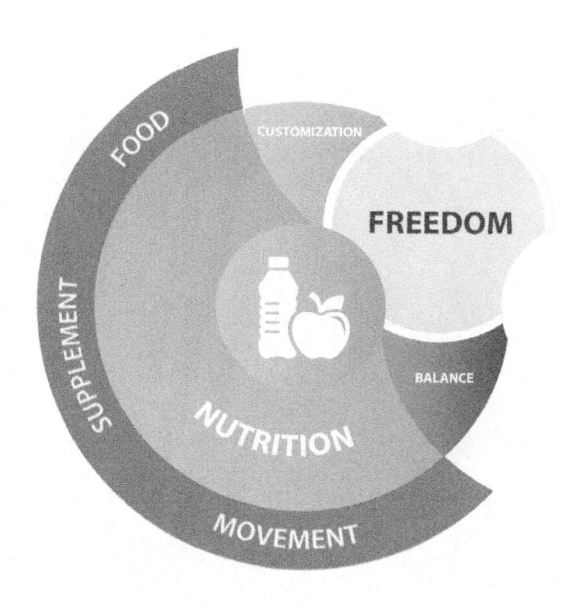

Nutrition is a critical component to healing, and a commonly misunderstood piece of the puzzle. Nutrition isn't as complicated as the experts would make you think it is. We're the only animal that feels the need to "learn" how to eat and nourish our bodies because we overcomplicate the eating process by commercializing food products rather than eating for our health.

Nature already provides complete nutrition to keep us energetic and healthy through whole foods. The confusion of what to eat is a negative result of advertising, prepackaged foods, and labeling processed foods as "natural" and "healthy" when they're anything but.

In this section, we'll demystify the unnecessarily complicated world of food, nutrition, and fitness so you better understand the right choices for you.

CHAPTER 9

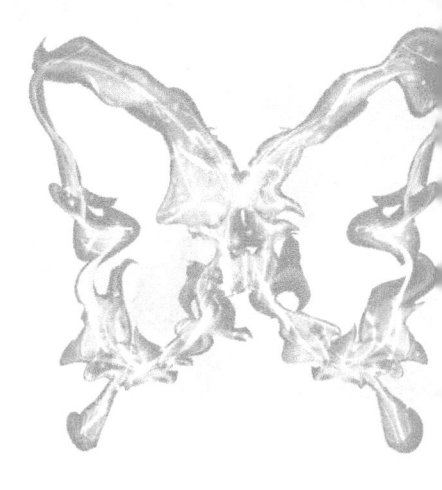

FOOD

"Let food be thy medicine and medicine be thy food."
- Hippocrates

Aida was 44 when she first started working with us. Her chief concerns were dermatomyositis (a skin condition that was nearly covering her face with dark patches, irritation, and swelling), lupus, low white blood cell count, inflammation, poor sleep, stress, and anxiety.

She was a mother and wife who was also caring for her own mother suffering from multiple ailments. Prior to working with us, she had worked with a medical doctor who had a program specifically for people with lupus. Aida followed the strict lupus recommended diet exactly as suggested. She attended all the program meetings, took the hundreds of dollars of program related supplements, and did everything that was recommended. After several months in the program, she wasn't seeing any results. She was told that she needed to get even more strict with her diet and to renew in the program for a second round. But even after doing exactly that, she still wasn't feeling any better and her lab results were getting worse.

We created a plan for Aida customized to her specific needs. Though there are similarities to people who have the same diagnosis, everyone is an individual and therefore each person requires some specific adjustments based on a variety of components.

Lupus, like any diagnosis, is simply a name for a collection of symptoms, it's not *the cause* of the symptoms. Which means, treating every person with a lupus diagnosis exactly the same way would be like treating every person with red hair and blue eyes the same way. Just because people with the same hair and eye color have a similar gene expression doesn't mean each of them is the same.

By following the far less restrictive diet we created for Aida, and doing the recommendations we gave her to reduce her anxiety and feel safe, within just a few days, Aida's body began to respond positively. A week later, her lab results showed that three foods that were highly recommended by the lupus specific diet she had been following previously, were foods that Aida's body had a strong aversion to and were actually creating more inflammation and symptoms for her.

At the three-month mark, Aida posted two pictures of herself (shown below). The first image is when she started in the Nourish Freedom Program and the other was taken just 12 weeks later. The shift in her skin condition and the reduction in swelling around her nose, eyes, and mouth was remarkable. Additionally, she was sleeping regularly and more soundly, her inflammation had reduced dramatically, and her anxiety had dropped.

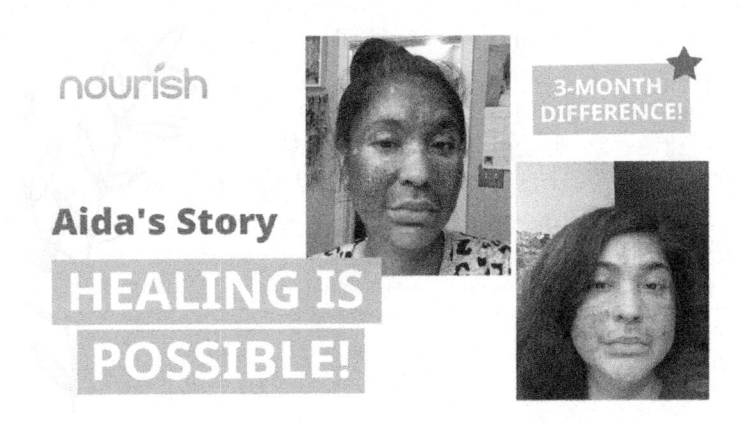

nourish

Aida's Story

HEALING IS POSSIBLE!

3-MONTH DIFFERENCE!

Six-months into the program, Aida's lab results also showed that her white blood cell count had improved, and all her other symptoms were getting better.

Her results improved because she was now following a health strategy designed for her individual needs physically, mentally, and emotionally. To hear her tell the rest of her story, you can go to www.Nourish123.com/case-studies.

Here's the thing: there's no perfect one-size-fits-all diet for everyone. There's not even a one-size-fits all diet for people in a specific category like lupus. There are some general guidelines, which we'll talk about in more detail shortly, but each person and situation is unique, and therefore needs to be treated as an individual.

It's why we encourage clients not to get locked into any one way to eat, and create the right diet for them to reach their health goals. We take into consideration data such as specific symptoms, age, cultural background, blood type, food likes and dislikes, lab results, medications they may have taken, and where they are on their unique healing trajectory.

Many practitioners have their clients follow a specific diet regimen such as paleo, AIP, vegan, or keto as if it's the answer for everyone. Again, from personal and professional experience, we've found that every person is a unique individual and their nutrition has to be dialed in and customized for them. We use about a dozen different factors when creating a nutrition strategy for a client, and we've found that the more comfortable a client is with their unique food plan the more likely they are to follow it and see results. A client who is stressed out about what they are eating, or terrified that they're "getting it wrong," is less likely to be able to relax, reduce stress, digest what they are eating, and absorb nutrients effectively.

The only things we're crystal clear on for every client when it comes to what not to eat are "toxic gluten" and dairy products because of the numerous studies supporting how inflammatory these food items are at some level to literally everyone who eats them.

"Toxic gluten" is anything that contains wheat, rye, barley, malt (and arguably oats). Breads, pasta, cereals, and baked goods are typically the most obvious culprits to contain toxic gluten. Dairy is anything that comes from an udder such as milk, cheese, butter, yogurt, and ice cream.

Now, just because there are studies that show how damaging gluten and dairy are to the gut and overall health, doesn't mean that everyone will agree (even some nutrition experts) that they need to be eliminated.

There are also thousands of studies proving without a doubt how harmful smoking is, though it's still a billion dollar industry. Essentially, if the gratification from consuming something is greater than the consequences, people will continue to participate in those activities even when they "know better."

After a dozen years, we have yet to work with someone who is doing better when eating gluten or dairy, and if you want to stop your symptoms and heal, we strongly recommend eliminating them from your diet.

Other than those two restrictions, we work with each client to create the right nutritional strategy for them.

Let's go deeper on why we don't recommend gluten or dairy.

Many clinical studies and books have been written on the negative effects of gluten and dairy on the body, and we've collected overwhelming anecdotal evidence working directly with clients that supports the removal of gluten and dairy.

One of our favorite clinical studies on gluten was performed by Justin Hollon, Elaine Leonard Puppa, Bruce Greenwald, Eric Goldberg, Anthony Guerrerio and Alessio Fasano titled "Effect of Gliadin on Permeability of Intestinal Biopsy Explants from Celiac Disease Patients and Patients with Non-Celiac Gluten Sensitivity."

The conclusion was that gliadin (a smaller component of toxic gluten) exposure induces an increase in intestinal permeability (leaky gut) in **all individuals,** regardless of whether or not they have celiac disease. https://www.ncbi.nlm.nih.gov/pmc/articles/PMC4377866/

To be clear, that means that literally *every single person* who was studied, even the ones who did not have celiac disease or any known gluten sensitivity at the time of the study, were negatively impacted by gluten when tested.

In addition to that, both dairy and wheat have similar enough proteins to human molecules where consuming them can result in cross-reactivity that leads to food autoimmunity and even autoimmune disorders. https://pubmed.ncbi.nlm.nih.gov/25599184/

This means that dairy often causes a similar negative reaction in the body as gluten because many times the protein in dairy is confused for being the same protein as the one found in gluten. This can trigger an autoimmune response, causing the body to attack itself, cause inflammation, and/or increase the chances of intestinal permeability (leaky gut.)

Ancient wheat had eight chromosomes. Today's wheat can have as many as 64 chromosomes with many of them being highly allergic.[1] In other words, when gluten and/or dairy are consumed, they can cause an immune response in which the immune system produces antibodies that not only react against the food but also against the body's own tissue. This is the very definition of autoimmune disease. When the immune system attacks the thyroid, it's called Hashimoto's. When the immune system attacks the gut, that's celiac disease. When it attacks the joints, it's known as rheumatoid arthritis. When the nerves are attacked, it's called multiple sclerosis. When the pigment of the skin is under attack, it's known as vitiligo. The list goes on and on.

As explained earlier, for an autoimmune disease to surface, three things must come together: a predisposition, leaky gut, and a trigger. Leaky gut, also known as intestinal permeability, is just as the name suggest, where the gut (small intestine) contents are "leaking" into the blood stream.

Leaking you ask? Yes. Actually leaking bits and pieces from the gut and small intestines into the blood, triggering alarms to go off in the system.

Facts About Your Gut

- Your intestinal epithelium wall is only one cell thick. So, there's essentially one cell separating what you consume from the outside world from your bloodstream.
- The surface area of your intestines is about 1/3 the size of a tennis court.
- 70% of your immune system is in your gut. (Yes! That's a lot and why a healthy balanced gut is critical to healing.)
- Your gut contains 3.3lbs to 4.4lbs of bacteria – more than the weight of your brain.

The more you understand about the gut, and why it could be leaking, the better your chances of creating the right healing solution for you.

The cells that make up the epithelium wall should be nice and tight like the "Normal Tight Junction" part of the diagram below shows. But because of insults to the epithelium wall, this allows partially digested food, toxins, and microbes to penetrate (or leak) and get into the bloodstream. This triggers inflammation and changes in the gut bacteria that could lead to issues within the digestive tract. Some common symptoms are bloating, gas, cramps, food sensitivities, and aches and pains.

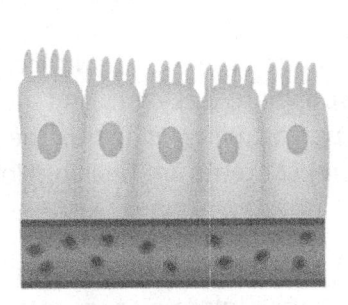

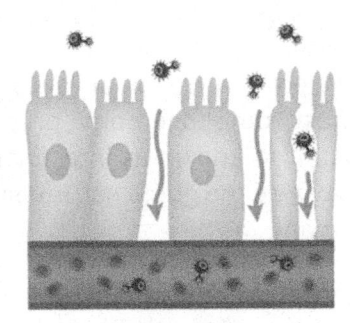

Normal Tight Junction   **Leaky and Inflamed**

Some of the insults that cause leaky gut are diet, lifestyle, medications, stress, dysbiosis, and toxins.

Now that you better understand leaky gut, let's dive further in to nutrition. Even though nutrition is specific and granular for each person, there are guidelines that we recommend to everyone.

- Avoid gluten and dairy. That goes double if you have any thyroid issues or celiac disease.
- Minimize highly processed foods. They contain little to no nutritional value and cause oscillations in glucose levels.
- If you eat animal protein, choose wild, grass fed, organic options. Check out Concentrated Animal Feeding Operation or CAFO for more details.
- Eat plenty of fruits and vegetables, especially green leafy ones and preferably organic.
- Shoot for 40+ grams of fiber per day. Gut bacteria make butyric acid from it, which is critical for optimal gut health.
- Eat beans, legumes, nuts, and seeds if you tolerate them. Pre-soaking before cooking helps digestibility.
- Eat raw fermented foods like sauerkraut and pickles. YAY! Probiotics.
- Keep sugar to an absolute minimum. Sugar keeps the immune system in a state of confusion, and confusion can lead to autoimmune disease.
- Keep caffeine to a minimum. It doesn't serve the adrenal glands, depletes B vitamins and blunts the absorption of iron.
- Keep alcohol to a minimum or not at all. It's a toxin, a diuretic, depletes B vitamins and makes for an unhappy liver.
- Drink clean water. Unfiltered tap water is not clean water. Clean water keeps your kidneys happy and helps prevent kidney stones.
- Get a powerful water filter. It's better to own a water filter than *be* a water filter. We recommend using a filter that uses both reverse osmosis and carbon block at the same time.
- Stay away from artificial flavors, colors, and other chemicals.
- Get good at reading ingredient lists on products and don't just look

at the marketing on the front of the product.

- Consider intermittent fasting. There are many health benefits to minimizing the amount of time your body spends digesting each day. Autophagy (the body's way of cleaning out damaged cells in order to regenerate newer healthier cells) is one of the most amazing benefits of fasting. So, give yourself at a minimum of 12 hours between your last meal of each day to your first meal of the next day.

- Use glass whenever possible. Plastic is a xenobiotic and an endocrine disruptor.[2]

- Avoid using pots/pans with Teflon. Be sure to watch the movie *Dark Waters* for all the details on why.

- Keep good oral hygiene. This is not necessarily nutrition, but the gums are a direct route into the blood stream for bacteria.

Chapter Takeaways

- Gluten and dairy are not your friends no matter who you are and even if you don't think you have any negative effects from eating them. Just because you don't notice, doesn't mean damage isn't happening at a cellular level.

- There is no perfect or one-size-fits-all diet. The right diet must be created for each person based on where they are in their health journey.

- Leaky gut is a trigger for autoimmune disease and chronic illness.

CHAPTER 10

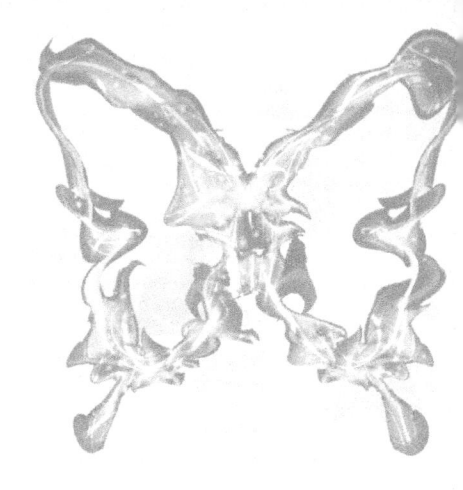

SUPPLEMENTS

In our industry, we see lots of oversupplementation. When clients begin working with us, they often have a cabinet full of supplements. Some are spending hundreds of dollars every month and taking 20-50 supplements a day! When you're full after taking your supplements, that's a problem.

Supplements absolutely have their place, but they're meant to *complement* a proper nutrition program, not be a substitute for one. In addition, many of the ingredients in the supplements we evaluate are often garbage which can cause problems of leaky gut and other negative reactions. Typically, you really do get what you pay for when it comes to supplements.

One of our jobs is to identify nutrient deficiencies/insufficiencies, and, if there are any, recommend food(s) that will give medicinal amounts of that nutrient.

Some nutrients are more challenging than others to get such as vitamin D. Few foods contain decent amounts of vitamin D, and really none have "medicinal amounts" in them, except maybe cod liver oil at 1,300 IU per tablespoon.

If a client's blood work comes back low for vitamin D, Anthony works with the client to determine *why*. Is there not enough intake of the nutrient? Is it not being absorbed properly? Is the body excreting it?

Only once he understands *the why* can he make a decision on how to proceed.

Vitamin D can be made in the skin from sun exposure. The sun's ultraviolet B rays hit cholesterol in the skin cells, which turns into vitamin D.

1,000 IU of vitamin D can be synthesized in adults by going outside in the summer or spring with at least 22% of the skin exposed and without sunscreen. This will vary with skin tone. The darker the skin, the more sun exposure is needed, since darker skin absorbs fewer ultraviolet B rays. Up to ten times more exposure is needed for the darkest skin.

The Recommended Dietary Allowance (RDA) is the average daily level of intake sufficient to meet the nutrient requirements of nearly all (97–98%) healthy individuals. If you look at the *% Daily Value* on food labels, the percentages are based on the bare minimum needed so you don't get disease. It is not based on "medicinal amounts" which means there's enough of the nutrient to cause a healing response.

So if you're only getting the RDA recommended amounts of nutrients each day, you won't be able to reach healing. You need much more than the minimum requirements. If you're not eating enough high quality foods or if you aren't absorbing enough of the nutrients from what you are eating, then you're going to struggle to get out of "crisis mode" and into "healing mode" as we talked about earlier.

If we had to pick one supplement to recommend, we'd go with a high-potency multivitamin. Why? Because there are about 30 vitamins and minerals we need to consume daily for all metabolic functions to run properly.

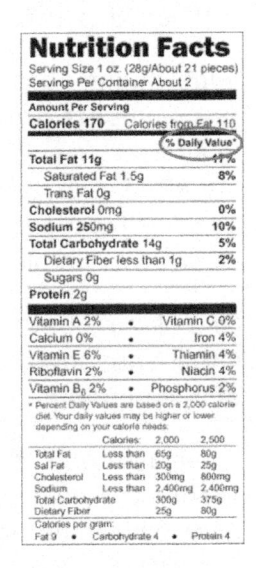

Below is a diagram showing biochemical pathways that are nutrient dependent. We included it to give you an idea of the sheer number of metabolic processes happening that are nutrient dependent.

Metabolic Metro Map

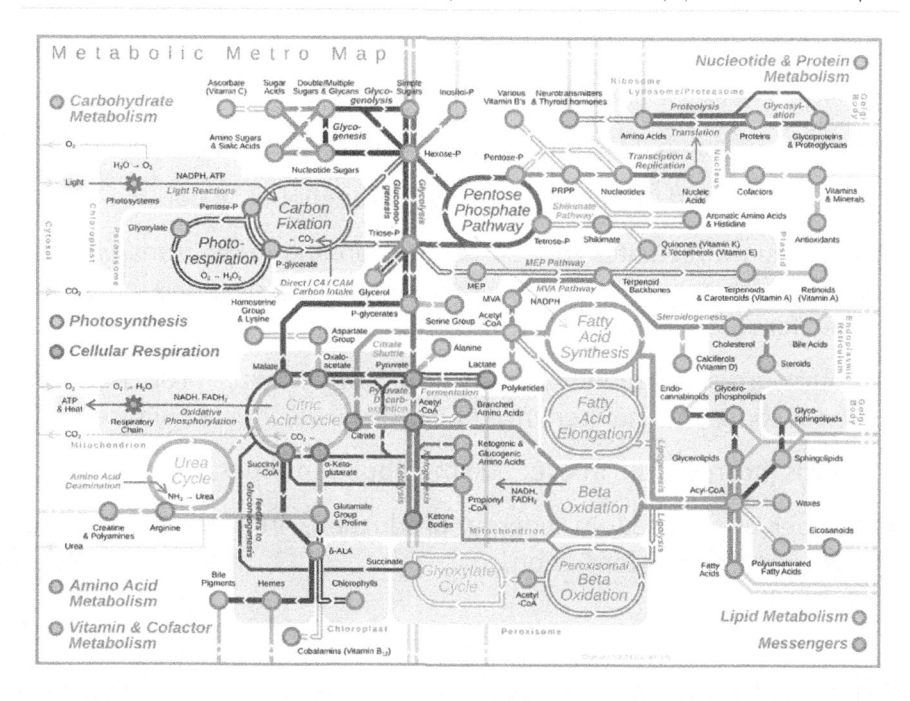

Here are some examples of what purpose certain vitamins and minerals perform:

- B vitamins are needed to extract energy from food, for healthy red blood cells and neurotransmitter formation.
- Vitamin C is a very potent antioxidant and plays an essential role in maintaining a strong immune system. Also necessary for iron absorption.
- Vitamin B12 is required for proper nerve function and to make red blood cells.
- Vitamin A is needed for good vision, immunity, and healthy skin.
- Vitamin D is required to form bone, healthy immune function, and it functions like a hormone throughout the body. It's also required for calcium absorption, enhances phosphorus absorption, and supports cardiovascular health.
- Vitamin E is an antioxidant and helps protect cells from free-radical damage.

- Vitamin K is needed to form blood clots and to spackle calcium onto the bones.
- Calcium is needed for muscle contraction and bone formation.
- Iron is required to transport oxygen throughout the body.
- Magnesium regulates muscle contraction and nerve transmission. It helps form teeth and bones and is needed in over 300 metabolic reactions.
- Potassium is needed for muscle contraction, proper nerve conduction, and maintenance of fluid and electrolyte balance.
- Zinc is incorporated in over 300 metabolic enzymes.
- Copper is needed in energy production, iron transport, and neurotransmitter formation.

Chapter Takeaways

- Supplements alone are not the answer. You cannot supplement your way to health. Choosing better quality food and making sure your body is capable of absorbing the nutrients in those foods is an important part of the transformational healing process.
- Don't guess; test for nutrient deficiencies/insufficiencies. There are certain nutrients which can be dangerous at high levels. More isn't necessarily better.
- A quality high-potency multivitamin is a good idea for many people. Make sure it isn't loaded with lots of fillers and other garbage or it will be a waste of money and won't help you get on the ideal healing path.

CHAPTER 11

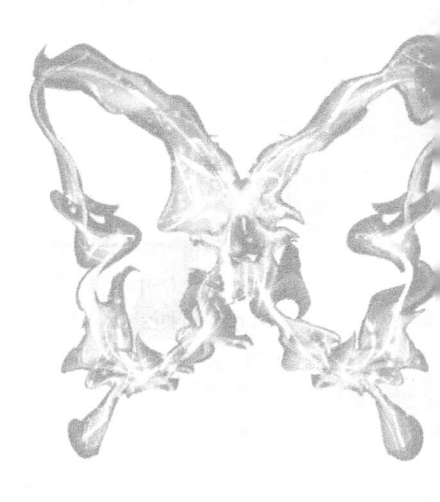

MOVEMENT

Move the body!

Exercise cleans up a lot of disorders, and it's never too late to start. Regular physical activity helps improve your overall health, fitness, and quality of life.

Check out all the amazing benefits to the right movement for you, as supported by MedlinePlus.gov:

- Helps control weight. Along with diet, exercise plays an important role in controlling weight and preventing obesity.

- Reduces the risk of heart diseases. Exercise strengthens the heart and improves circulation. The increased blood flow raises the oxygen levels in your body, which can lower risk of heart diseases such as high cholesterol, coronary artery disease, and heart attack. Regular exercise can also lower blood pressure and triglyceride levels.

- Helps the body manage blood sugar and insulin levels. This can cut down the risk for metabolic syndrome and type 2 diabetes. And if you already have one of those diseases, exercise can help you to manage it.

- Helps you quit smoking. Exercise may make it easier to quit by reducing your cravings and withdrawal symptoms. It can also help limit the weight you might gain when you stop smoking.

- Improves mental health and mood. During exercise, the body releases chemicals that can improve mood and make you feel more relaxed. This can help you deal with stress and reduce your risk of depression.
- Helps keep thinking, learning, and judgment skills sharp as you age. Exercise stimulates the body to release proteins and other chemicals that improve the structure and function of your brain.
- Strengthens bones and muscles. It can also slow bone density loss. Doing muscle-strengthening activities can help you increase or maintain your muscle mass and strength.
- Reduces risk of some cancers, including colon, breast, uterine, and lung cancer.
- Improves sleep. Exercise can help you to fall asleep faster and stay asleep longer.
- Reduces PMS issues such as bloating, gas, cramping, clotting, water retention, nausea, and excessive or heavy bleeding.
- Improves sexual health and may increase sexual arousal.
- Increases chances of living longer. Studies show that physical activity can reduce risk of dying early from the leading causes of death, like heart disease and some cancers.

We're fans of walking, resistance training, and yoga. The client's goals, resources, and interests determine the type, duration, intensity, and frequency we recommend.

Anthony is a Certified Personal Trainer and a body builder. From both professional and personal experience, he prefers to see clients do some level of cardiovascular activity and resistance training. For those with osteopenia or osteoporosis, resistance training is critical to building strong bones. Taking calcium/vitamin K supplements isn't enough. There needs to be an element of weight bearing exercise. Even just climbing stairs, can increase bone density.

Movement is incredibly important in the process of healing, but the right movement for you based on where you are in your healing journey is most important. In other words, you want to make sure your adrenal glands and nervous system aren't being overworked, which leads to long recovery times, and can keep you from getting out of crisis mode and into healing mode.

In addition, people can get out of balance or obsessed with exercising, thinking they can "outwork" their condition or illness. Exercise technically engages the fight-or-flight response and like everything else, needs to be dialed in for each person to transform their health.

It's important to be mindful that if you are already in a chronic state of stress, the type of exercise you're doing may need to be adjusted. Again, there's no one-size-fits-all workout, either.

Movement & Healing

One of the preconditions of well-being is being able to feel "at home" in your body.

We can purposefully use movement and rest not only to connect with and feel at home in our body, but also to facilitate healing with the body. We can cultivate transformational healing by getting to know the various styles of movement and rest available, so we can care for and nourish ourselves each day in the ways that bring balance and enjoyment to our system.

Most people are familiar with dynamic forms of movement like walking, hiking, dancing, stretching, and yoga flows. Dynamic movement is any activity that involves continuous physical movement and heightened breathing. It helps to activate the systems of the body, encouraging:

- Healthy circulation of blood, lymph, and oxygen through the body.
- Release of excess energy and/or pent-up emotions.
- Elevation of energy and/or mood.

And movement is still happening even when we're static! Our thoughts are moving, our blood is moving, our breath is moving, and it is here within this "static movement," we can connect to Self.

Static forms of movement (also known as restorative movement [1,2,3,4]) include restorative yoga, meditation sessions, breathing exercises, daydreaming, and journaling. Static movement helps calm and relax the systems of the body, encouraging:

- Relaxation of physical, mental, emotional, and biochemical energy patterns.
- Gentle massage and stimulation of internal organs to improve function.
- Grounding and balancing of energy and/or mood.

When we learn how to use various forms of movement to bring enjoyment and balance to our everyday lives, we start to tap into the potential to create serious change in our health and Selves.

Daily Movement

When it comes to daily movement for a body that's experiencing chronic symptoms like fatigue, anxiety, digestive distress, and hormone imbalances, it's important to be aware of not over-extending and pushing too far too soon. As we've already mentioned, this will add unnecessary strain to the adrenal glands and other systems of the body.

Instead, focus on cultivating relaxation and choose activities that help you feel relaxed and at peace. Some great examples of relaxing movement that are ideal for daily use include:

- Walking for at least 30 minutes every day, especially out in nature.
- Enjoying a restorative yoga pose while being mindful of the breath for three to five minutes each day.
- Taking time in stillness to be with Self and the breath, for at least 60 seconds every single day.

You can set yourself up for success by choosing activities that feel accessible and achievable for you on any given day. Does walking for 15 minutes feel like too much today? Choose to walk for five minutes instead. If that feels too much, simply get out of the house and enjoy some fresh air and sun on your face for a few minutes while you check in with Self and be with your breath for a few moments. This is also a great way to get in some valuable vitamin D, too! Any action you take is a win!

Tools for Balance

We can use our breath and our bodies to help facilitate physical, mental, and emotional balance and relaxation.

Exploring the technique of Alternate Nostril Breathing [5] (also known as nadi shodhana pranayama) is one of the best ways to bring balance to our physical state, our mental state, and our emotional state. It's been proven to lower stress as well as help improve blood pressure biomarkers and cardiovascular function. It helps to strengthen the awareness of and sensitivity to our breath, and balances the energies of the left and right brain hemispheres.

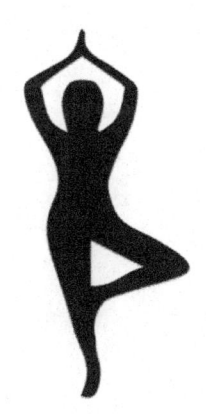

Balancing positions like the well-known "prayer pose" or "tree pose" in yoga, help develop the function of the cerebellum, which is the part of the brain that controls how the body moves; they help improve muscle coordination and posture while training the body to embrace stillness in static forms of movement.

If you're ever feeling off-balance emotionally and/or mentally, you can move into a balancing posture and connect with your breath for just a few minutes to feel a significant shift in how the body, mind, and emotions are showing up.

Chapter Takeaways

- Our bodies were not designed to be sedentary. Movement is critical for transformational healing, even if it's just a walk around the block.

- It's never too late to start moving the body. Even a 60 second exercise can get you rolling. Why not start right now?

- Movement has a long list of health benefits and every one of them can be the tipping point to shifting you from the poor health trajectory to the ideal one!

CHAPTER 12

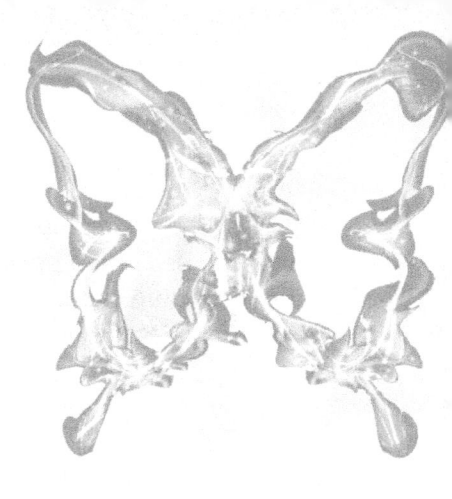

SLEEP

You might be wondering why we added a chapter on sleep in the "Nutrition Section" of this book. It's because sleep is critical to movement, repair, processing, absorption, and the support of all the systems necessary for optimal health. Sleep is a process we keep tabs on with our clients because it's so important. Not only how many hours each night they're getting, but also things like:

- Do you dream?
- Do you drool in your sleep?
- Do you fall asleep easily and stay asleep?
- Is there a particular time you consistently wake up during the night?
- Do you feel rested and refreshed when it's time to get up?

Sleep is essential to the body. It's when the body repairs, when the immune system is most active and growth hormone is released. Our heart rate and breathing slow down, body temperature falls, muscles twitch, and our brain waves change.

Sleep is regulated by circadian rhythms, which are synchronized by the hypothalamus, located in the brain. Circadian rhythms are physical, mental, and behavioral changes that follow a 24-hour cycle. For example, cortisol should be highest in the morning and lowest in the evening. The production of melatonin is ramped up at night and switches to serotonin production when it begins to get light out. Most of the melatonin production takes place in the pineal gland, located in the brain. Melatonin is a hormone that helps regulate our sleep-wake cycle.

Research at Stamford University has shown that a lack of sleep or insomnia is detrimental to stem cell function in the body. A reduction of night sleep to four hours (instead of eight) decreases the ability of stem cells to migrate by nearly 50%, while proper seven-to-eight-hour sleep cycles do the opposite and renew the quantitative and qualitative indices of circulating stem cells. And only two hours of restorative sleep normalize the functional parameters of stem cells.[1]

We do not have a TV in our bedroom and do not recommend doing anything that is too stimulating to the brain within an hour of going to bed, like playing with a smart phone or anything else with a white screen. The stimulation and blue light emitted from your phone, TV, or other devices, restrains the production of melatonin. It can also reduce the total amount of REM (rapid eye movement) sleep and compromises alertness the next morning. So, if anything, read a book.

Because of modern lifestyles, stress, and advancements in technology, people are sleeping less than they were a century ago. Sleeping less than seven hours a night, is associated with chronic conditions like diabetes, obesity, and heart disease, and it can decrease lifespan.

Chapter Takeaways

- Eight+ hours of sleep per night is important.
- Watching TV or playing on your phone right before bed are not recommended.
- Melatonin is the hormone responsible for sleep.

PART 3

SCIENCE

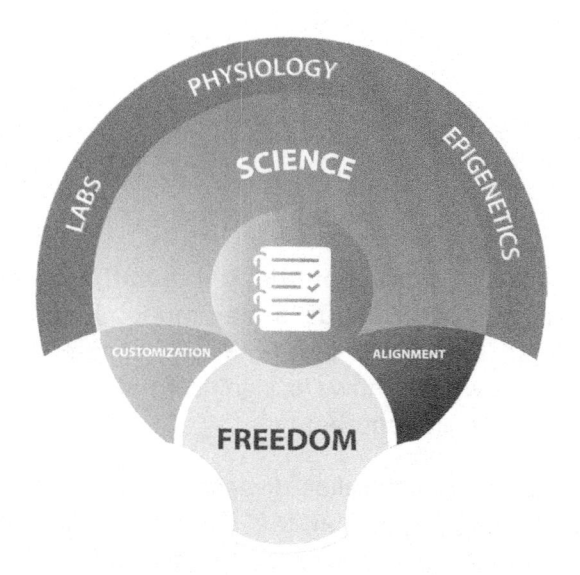

In this section, we'll show you the science behind the fear, thoughts, and beliefs that are going on in your body, in your cells and tissues; how they've been impacting your hormone balances, immune system response, and ability to heal; and why your symptoms are appearing and potentially getting worse, even though you're trying so hard to find the right pieces to your healing puzzle.

We'll also dive into the world of epigenetics and show what triggers genes to express health or disease, and explain more about the "Science Section" of our healing model.

Genesis of CoMorbidities

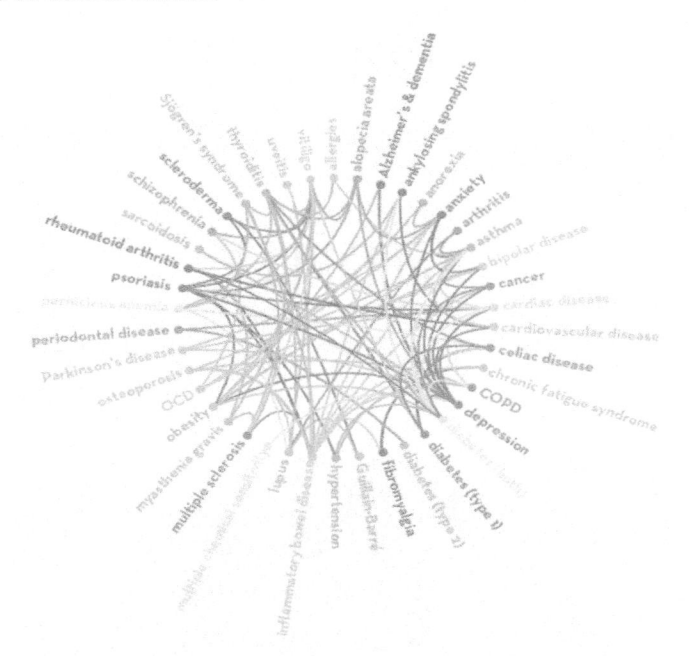

This diagram, which is framed on the wall of Anthony's office, shows the correlation between various autoimmune diseases and other chronic illnesses. Each spoke of the wheel represents a published study in MEDLINE which shows a significant statistical relationship between one disease and another.

Kirstin was diagnosed with celiac disease, and later diagnosed with Hashimoto's. When you look at the diagram, notice that the line connecting to celiac, also connects to thyroiditis, which includes Hashimoto's.

We believe at the rate this country's going, every health issue is going to be connected to autoimmune disease at some level. Recently, all three types of diabetes were reclassified as autoimmune, as was heart disease. Understanding what autoimmune disease is, how to protect yourself (and loved ones) from it, and how it impacts the body is critical, because very soon everyone will be impacted by it in some way, directly or indirectly.

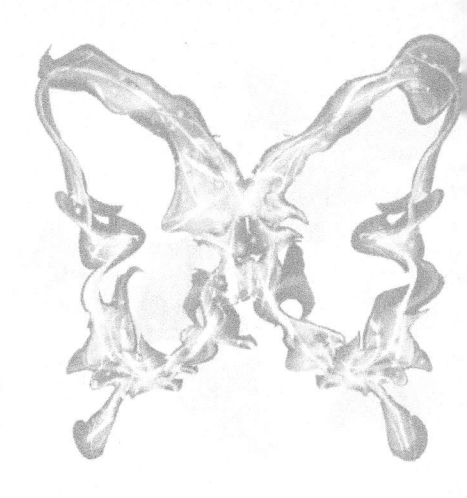

CHAPTER 13

ADRENAL FUNCTION

Let's chat about adrenal glands. The adrenals are responsible for our stress response and how stress impacts overall physiology. They essentially tie together all the systems in the body, so if they are stressed out, other bodily functions are also impacted, making them pretty important to overall health.

Whether or not you believe the stress in your life is justified or valid, it is not serving your health in a positive way. The adrenal glands are glands that sit on top of the kidneys and are about the size of a walnut. They produce various stress hormones, and they also produce sex or steroid hormones like DHEA. Looking at the cross section of an adrenal gland, certain layers produce certain hormones and chemicals. For now, let's focus on the stress response.

Adrenal Gland

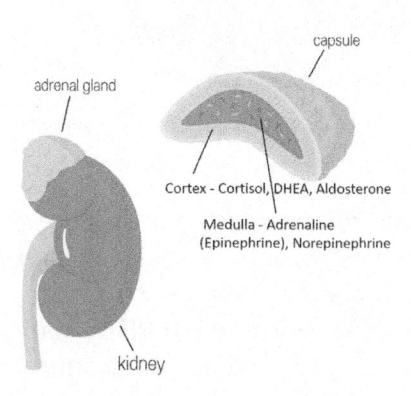

capsule
adrenal gland
Cortex - Cortisol, DHEA, Aldosterone
Medulla - Adrenaline (Epinephrine), Norepinephrine
kidney

The chemicals that put the body into a fight-or-flight state are cortisol, adrenaline, and epinephrine. Cortisol has a bad reputation, though it actually plays a very important role in energy production and has anti-inflammatory properties. So, cortisol isn't all bad. It's actually healthy to have a short-term stress response, but when the perceived threat is over, the stress response should go away. If it doesn't and the adrenals are constantly producing cortisol, that's not optimal.

Here's the cascade of events:

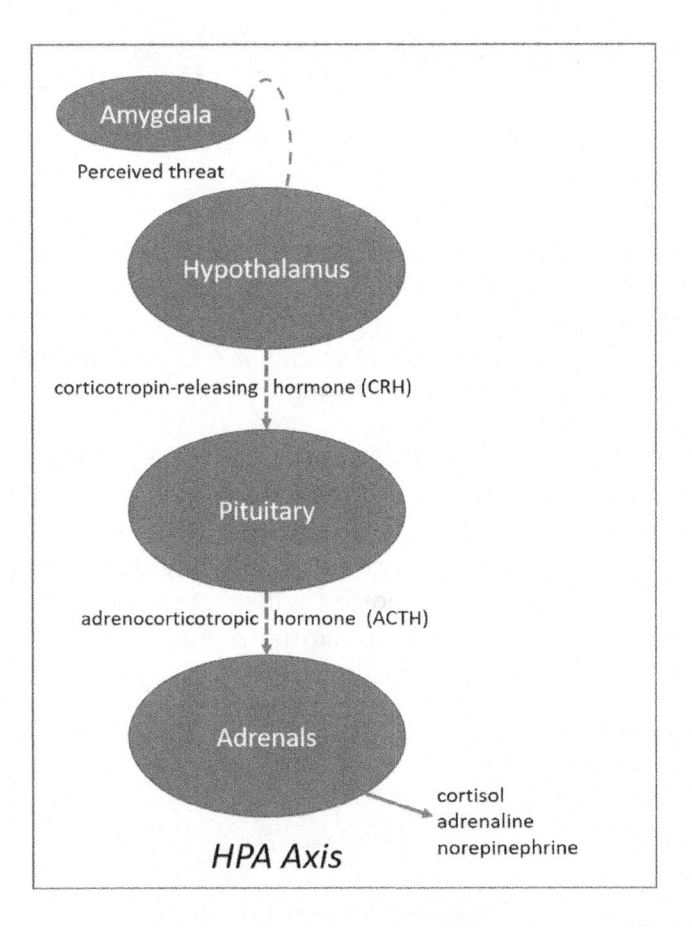

```
            Amygdala
         Perceived threat
              │
              ▼
          Hypothalamus
              │
  corticotropin-releasing hormone (CRH)
              │
              ▼
           Pituitary
              │
  adrenocorticotropic hormone (ACTH)
              │
              ▼
           Adrenals
                      → cortisol
                        adrenaline
          HPA Axis      norepinephrine
```

When the amygdala, which is part of the brain, perceives something as threatening, dangerous, or unsafe, it signals another part of the brain called the hypothalamus, which creates a hormone called Corticotropin-Releasing Hormone (CRH). That signals the pituitary gland, also part of the brain, to produce a hormone called

Adrenocorticotropic Hormone (ACTH). This signals the adrenals that there's danger and it's unsafe. The adrenals then produce cortisol, adrenaline, and norepinephrine. This cascade of events is known as the hypothalamic-pituitary-adrenal axis or HPA axis and triggers a change in blood flow in the body and the brain. Instead of the blood being mostly in the visceral tissues (lungs, heart, and the organs of the digestive, excretory, reproductive, and circulatory systems), the "threat" causes blood flow to preferentially go to the arms and legs. Why? So, the body is more prepared to run or fight. In the brain, blood flow shifts from the part that makes logical decisions to the one that makes more reactive decisions.

That's why when the stress response kicks in and stress hormones are flowing, you will typically feel more "triggered," short-tempered, and reactive, and why it may feel more difficult to think clearly and rationally, and govern your emotions.

Biomarkers on a blood chemistry screen can identify optimal adrenal function, adrenal hypofunction, or adrenal stress. Symptoms include, but aren't limited to chronic fatigue, irritability, decreased immune function, low blood pressure, glucose dysregulation, anxiety, poor concentration/memory, hormone dysfunction, and PMS. Adrenal issues can cause immune, hormone, and metabolic breakdown.

A part of our central nervous system (CNS) called the autonomic nervous system (ANS) maintains homeostasis (balance) and controls all our unconscious functions like digestion, breathing, heart rate, and blood pressure. The ANS is broken up into two different parts: the sympathetic, also known by its catchy name, "fight-or-flight." Think of it as an "accelerator" because it amps you up. It's the part of the autonomic nervous system that increases heart rate, breathing, sweating, and pupil dilation. The second part is the parasympathetic, which is the exact opposite of the sympathetic. Its catchy name is "rest-and-digest." Think of it as the "brakes" because it slows you down.

Both are important, and you are never in either one 100%. It's about balance. Being in fight-or-flight from time to time is okay. It actually makes us resilient and can save our lives. There's an enormous difference between being in a chronic vs. acute state of fight-or-flight. Anthony used to work in Manhattan and sometimes worked late nights. When he was walking from work to Grand Central Station to catch the Metro North to go home, if he saw a suspicious character roaming the streets, the fight-or-flight response would kick in.

When there is a perceived threat and we feel unsafe, the fight-or-flight response should be activated. That's expected, and it's how the body was designed to work. Then, a few minutes or so after the threat is gone, our bodies should go back into a rest-and-digest state. Stress, from time to time, is okay. We just don't want to live there. It's not optimal to be in a chronic state of fight-or-flight. Many people don't realize that they're living there because they're in it all the time. The body wasn't designed for long periods of this level of stress response.

When we sense danger or feel unsafe, whether we're stressed from work, finances, health, relationships, or kids, the sympathetic nervous system comes online. The body doesn't differentiate between types of stress. A stressful thought can actually kick off the whole HPA axis cascade mentioned earlier and cause all sorts of havoc, the same as actual physical danger.

Emotional stress is one form of stress. There's also physical stress (injury, infections, surgery) as well as chemical stress (medications, toxins, heavy metals). Working out has many benefits and is an important part of transformational healing. As we've mentioned, it's still a stressor on the system because it falls in line with your sympathetic response kicking in where heart rate, breathing, and stress hormones are increased. Though after working out, a healthy body should flip into a rest-and-digest state within a relatively short period of time.

When we feel safe, those feelings create a flood of 1,400 biochemical changes that promote growth and repair.[1] When we find that we're in patterns of feeling hurt, anger, stress, jealousy, rage, competition, or frustration, it causes a release of about 1,200 chemicals into the body. This chemical dump lasts about 90 seconds to two minutes.[2]

Later in Chapter 18: Epigenetics, we're going to go deeper into how these chemical dumps impact you on a genetic level, and how the chemistry our body creates from experiences that happen in our physical reality or from thought alone can impact genetic expression. It's pretty amazing stuff.

By the time people meet with us for the first time, they've typically been dealing with their issues, diseases, and diagnosis for many years and their identity is often strongly tied to their poor health trajectory. Their adrenal pattern is usually in a chronic state, so their adrenal glands are constantly shooting hormones like adrenaline and cortisol, keeping them in a high state of adrenal stress, keeping them from shifting out of "crisis mode" and into "healing mode."

Over time, the adrenal glands can become depleted because of the constant production of stress hormones and chemicals. When the adrenal glands are depleted, it's known as "adrenal dysfunction." When this happens, just imagine the adrenal glands waving white flags because they're too exhausted to produce hormones and just give up.

It's at this point when all havoc breaks loose in the body causing symptoms such as severe hormone imbalance, extreme fatigue, depression, foggy brain, impossible belly fat, poor sleep patterns, constant irritation and frustration, hopelessness, and a litany of other symptoms and disease.

Interestingly, you can become addicted to this chemical cocktail produced by the body, even when that chemical cocktail is doing more harm than good, just like a drug addict looking for drugs to get their short-term fix.

There is an emotion connected to every experience, and emotions are the chemical residue of those experiences. If your body is addicted to stress hormones, you will use your perception of the world around you and your emotional connection to those perceptions to keep triggering experiences that release specific chemical cocktails.

Dr. Joe Dispenza in his book *Becoming Supernatural: How Common People Are Doing the Uncommon,* he uses the following example to explain this cycle:

You might use your boss to reaffirm your addiction to judgment, your coworkers to reaffirm your addiction to competition, your friends to reaffirm your addiction to suffering, your enemies to reaffirm your addiction to hatred. You might use your parents to reaffirm your addiction to guilt, your Facebook feed to reaffirm your addiction to insecurity, the news to reaffirm your addiction to anger, your ex to reaffirm your addiction to resentment, or your relationship with money to reaffirm your addiction to lack and scarcity.

When we feel danger or feel unsafe, in addition to adrenal glands coming online and producing cortisol and adrenaline, we also get a spike in glucose because the body mobilizes stored forms of glucose called glycogen so we have the energy to fight or flee the danger. Some of our clients' glucose markers are above optimal (more on optimal versus normal ranges later in Chapter 15 when we discuss labs) when they start working with us because they're in a chronic state of stress. Because of this, the body downregulates (reduces or suppresses) the immune system, sex hormone production, and signals genes to create disease.

Chapter Takeaways

- When we are in survival mode producing lots of stress hormones, we use an enormous amount of energy, which can take away from creativity, growth, repair, healing, and returning to balance.

- Our bodies were designed to be in a stressed state for only a short time.

- Your body doesn't care if stress is caused from something in your physical reality, in your imagination, or through your thoughts. It doesn't matter if the threat is valid or perceived. Stress will always produce corresponding chemistry.

- Stress chemicals become addicting just like an additive drug, cigarettes, or sugar. When you become addicted to the feelings produced by stress chemicals, you can behave the same as a drug addict looking to get their fix.

- Chronic stress downregulates the immune system and hormone production, and signals genes to express that cause disease.

CHAPTER 14

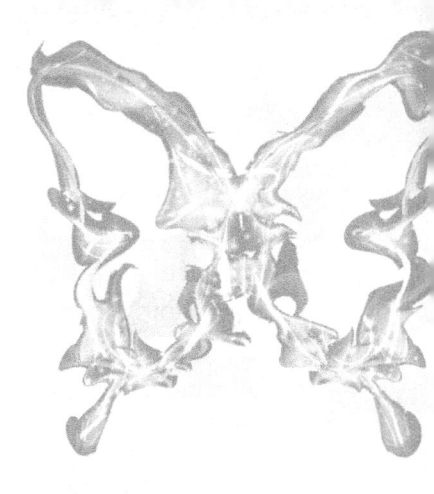

THE IMMUNE SYSTEM

Your immune system has two jobs:

1. To protect you from viruses, bacteria, pathogens, parasites, microbes, etc.
2. To help you heal.

When you cut yourself or when you bang your toe, there's a reason why it causes inflammation. The body is rushing oxygen, blood, nutrients, and immune cells to the damage area, so the immune system can come in, clean it up, and repair it. As you learned in the last chapter on adrenal function, being in a sustained chronic level of stress downregulates our immune system, which slows healing and protecting. It also causes the suppression of hormone production, and the expression of certain genes.

Here's why: Let's say you have a bacterial infection. You go outside and a saber-toothed tiger starts to chase you. What's more important to your body in that moment, escaping the danger or fighting the bacterial infection? Right, escaping the danger is more important than fighting an infection because survival is the most important thing. And if the saber-toothed tiger eats you, the bacterial infection is her problem now.

Also, before menopause kicks in, half of your sex hormone production is from the ovaries, the other half is produced by the adrenal glands. So, if the adrenals are already under stress from feeling unsafe and in danger, it's going to impact sex hormone production because survival is the top priority to your body. This means your body is going to focus on producing survival related chemistry, before creating or balancing hormones.

Men go through their own version of menopause too (called andropause) where the testes shut down the production of sex hormones. For both women and men, as sex hormone production slows from the sex organs, the adrenal glands become responsible to produce 100% of sex hormones. Think about it; if your adrenals are already taxed from stress when coming into menopause or andropause, now you're putting an extra burden on them to make up the difference in sex hormone production, it's going to cause you to hit a wall.

This is why you see so many women and men struggling as their hormone production begins to shift, sometimes as early as 30 years old as they move towards menopause and andropause. Energy drops, memory becomes a challenge, the ability to manage stress goes down, thyroid function becomes an issue, joint pain increases, belly fat appears, hair loss starts, libido drops, and depression becomes less manageable.

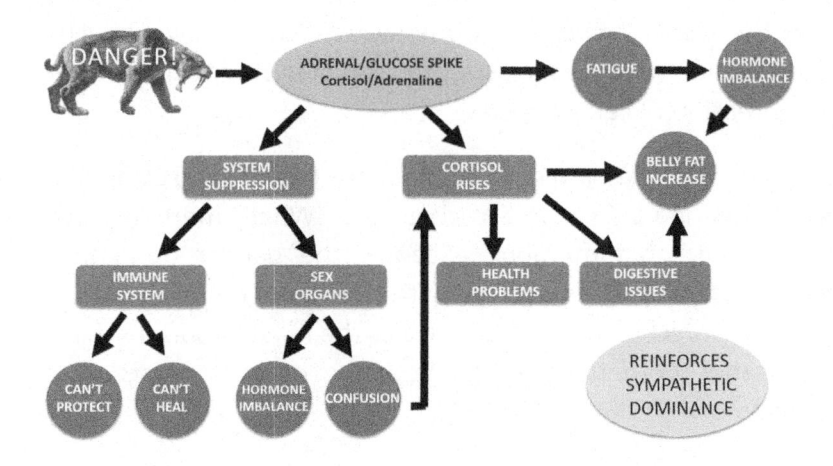

This diagram pulls it all together. Danger (or the perception of danger) represented by the saber-toothed tiger causes the adrenals to produce stress hormones. This causes a spike in glucose and a downregulation of the immune system and hormone production. So, the immune system's healing and protecting properties get lowered and sex hormone production decreases, which leads to health problems like fatigue, anxiety, and hormone imbalance.

Hormone imbalance leads to more cortisol release because it's causing more stress. And, as we already discussed, when the adrenals are already depleted from stress, putting more stress on them will simply lead to even more health problems, digestive issues, and belly fat.

When weight gain is mostly in the midsection, we've found that it's typically because of sustained chronic stress. As discussed in Lori's story in Chapter 6: Hidden Drivers, excess belly fat is often a way for the body to create a protective layer around one of the most vulnerable areas of the body, especially for women. Weight gain that is distributed all over the body we've found to be more often due to imbalances of sex hormones like estrogen and progesterone. This cascade puts the body in a chronic sympathetic state. And we weren't designed for that.

As pointed out by Dr. Joe Dispenza in his book, *You Are the Placebo: Making Your Mind Matter,* when living in chronic survival mode with the stress response turned on all the time, constantly bracing for worst-case scenarios, the mind can really only focus on three things:

1. The physical body. Am I okay?
2. The environment. Is it safe?
3. Time. How long is this threat going to be hanging over me?

By being constantly focused on these three things, it changes our ability to connect with ourselves spiritually, lowers awareness, and decreases mindfulness. All of which are critical to healing.

82 | Transformational Healing

Look at the figure below. Physiologically, having a sense of belonging, connectedness, community, and purpose, and being part of "a tribe" silences inflammatory genes and expresses antiviral gene expression.[1]

By sense of belonging, we don't mean how many Facebook friends or Instagram followers you have.

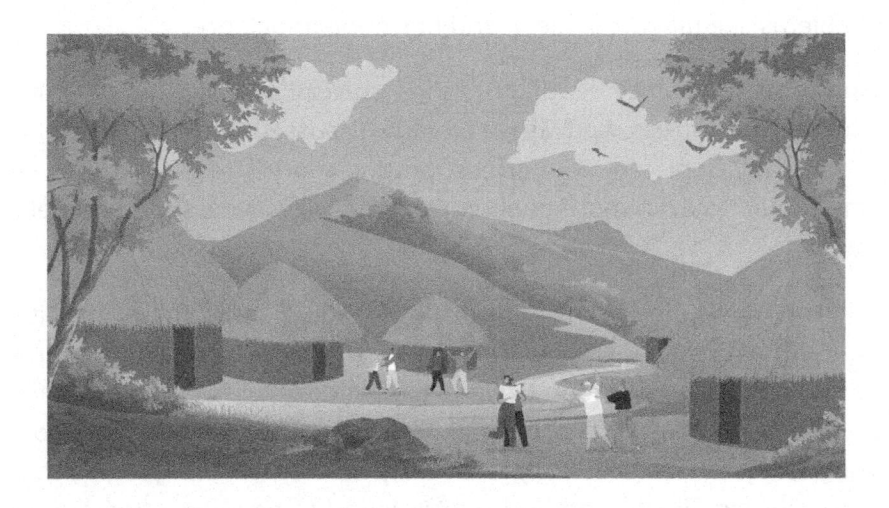

In the figure below, physiologically, when we don't have a sense of belonging, when we are not connected, when we are lonely, this expresses inflammatory genes and silences antiviral gene expression.[1]

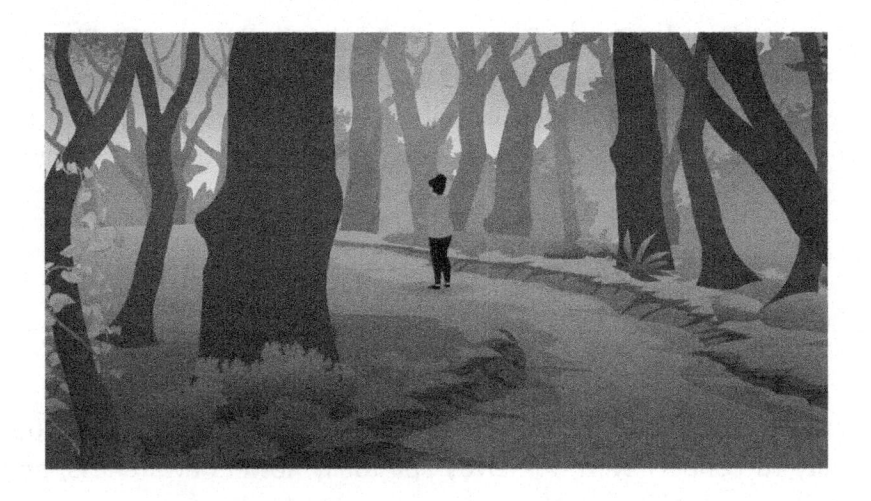

Chapter Takeaways

- The immune system not only protects you, but helps you heal.

- A sense of belonging, connectedness, and purpose silences inflammatory genes and expresses antiviral gene expression.

- Without a sense of belonging, connectedness, and purpose, this expresses inflammatory genes and silences antiviral gene expression.

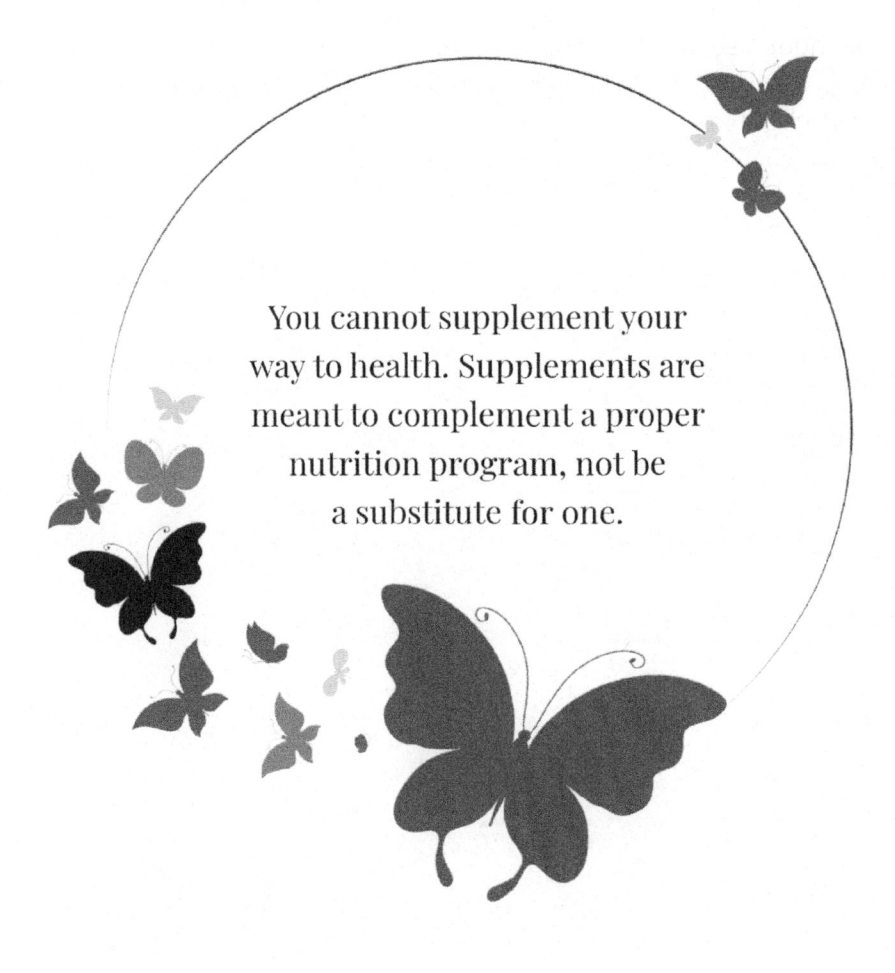

> You cannot supplement your way to health. Supplements are meant to complement a proper nutrition program, not be a substitute for one.

CHAPTER 15

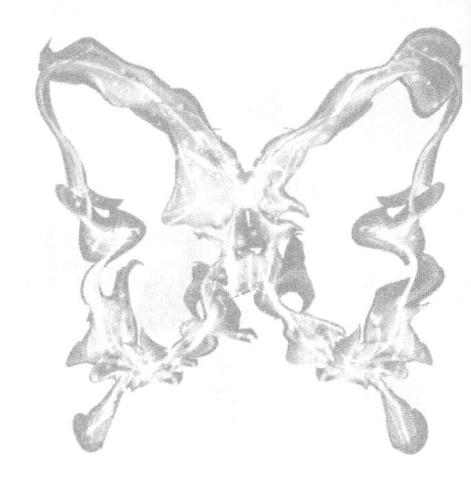

LABS

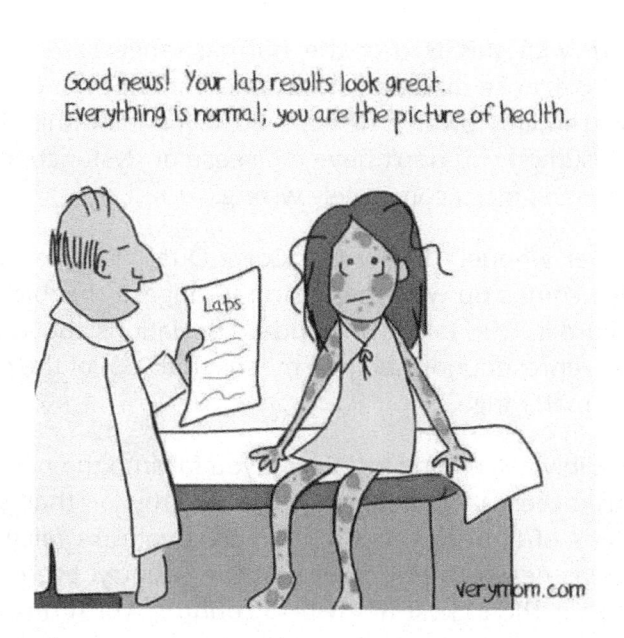

> Good news! Your lab results look great. Everything is normal; you are the picture of health.
>
> verymom.com

Anthony nerds out with our clients when discussing their labs with them. He loves to teach and educate them on what the markers suggest, so they can discuss them further with their doctor. The goal of a lab meeting is to give the client a clear understanding of what the results mean and a clear path on what can be done to help them feel better and so their biomarkers show improvement when they do labs in the future.

We find that symptoms almost always precede what the labs indicate, which explain why so many of our clients who are suffering with a bucket load of symptoms say, "My doctor says my labs are normal." This creates a false sense that "everything is ok" and doesn't address the very real symptoms the client is experiencing. Let's talk about why that happens.

Many practitioners use conventional lab reference ranges (normal range) to interpret lab results on a blood chemistry screen. They compare a biomarker result to the "normal range" to determine whether or not the results are normal or abnormal to fit patients/clients in a particular disease pattern or pathology.

The problem with this is that the normal ranges are designed to identify and diagnose diseased states and pathology and not show if someone is trending towards disease. So, if you fall within the normal range, it's assumed you don't have a disease or dysfunction. And this assumption is too often completely wrong.

Have you ever wondered how Lab Corp, Quest Diagnostics, or any other US lab comes up with their normal ranges? This blew us away when we heard it. They take two standard deviations above and below the mean to represent normal. This means that 95% of the population is in the "normal" range.

This is incredibly misleading because if you fall into the normal range, that doesn't necessarily mean you are healthy or that you aren't showing signs of ill health. It simply means you are falling into the same range as nearly everyone else in the country! Even worse, the United States is the sickest first-world country, which means the lab companies are basing your "normal" results on the results of the average person in the US. Further, if the lab marker is higher or lower than the normal range, that means you fall in the outlying 2.5% percentile! These high and low markers are typically diseases states. This isn't okay.

For our clients, we focus on evidence based "optimal ranges", which are more useful and not just based on averages. We also look for patterns in blood work that identify dysfunction of a particular organ, gland, or system as well as nutrient deficiencies/insufficiencies. This gives clients an opportunity to discuss these findings with their doctor so they can identify and deal with issues before they become disease.

Functional vs. Pathological

Medicine and health care are undergoing a paradigm shift. We are seeing more and more demand to interpret from a more holistic rather than mechanistic or reductionistic perspective. Here are the differences between a pathological view of the body and a functional view of the body.[1]

Pathological View	Functional View
1. The body is viewed as a machine composed of separate systems reduced into its constituent parts.	1. The body is viewed as a dynamic and complex interconnected system of mind, body, and emotions.
2. Emphasis is placed on the identification of disease or pathology tissue change.	2. Emphasis is placed on the identification of areas of imbalance or dysfunction in normal physiology.
3. Diagnosis is extremely specialized.	3. Diagnosis integrates data from many different systems and methods.
4. Treatment is based on reducing symptoms.	4. Treatment addresses the underlying cause of dysfunction.
5. Major focus is spent on how the patient is doing	5. Major focus is spent on both subjective and

based on charts, statistics, and test results that are measured against a statistical "normal population".	objective information gathering based on a concept of optimal physiological function.
6. Relies on late-stage development of disease as a marker.	6. Allows for early prediction of dysfunction.
7. Health is measured as an absence of disease. As long as you do not have a disease, you are considered healthy.	7. Health is measured along a wellness continuum which is a spectrum moving from health to disease. Intervention can be made at every stage of the spectrum to restore and/or improve health and wellness.

It's also interesting how many different types of labs some practitioners run on their patients. Some of our clients say their recent round of labs cost $5,000-$10,000 dollars. OUCH! Their doctors run blood, saliva, urine, genetic, hair, stool, and just about any other type of test available, looking for a "magic unicorn" answer rather than focusing on the basics, which is where most all of the answers are when you know what to look for. We prefer blood chemistry. It may not be the sexiest, but it's been validated, around for many years, and internationally recognized. And not only is it much more cost effective, it reveals tons of valuable information when used effectively.

Chapter Takeaways

- Normal is not optimal.

- Conventional lab interpretation has an emphasis on disease or pathology and is based on reducing symptoms. Functional lab interpretation has an emphasis on imbalance or dysfunction and is based on identifying root cause.

- Running more and more labs is not the answer.

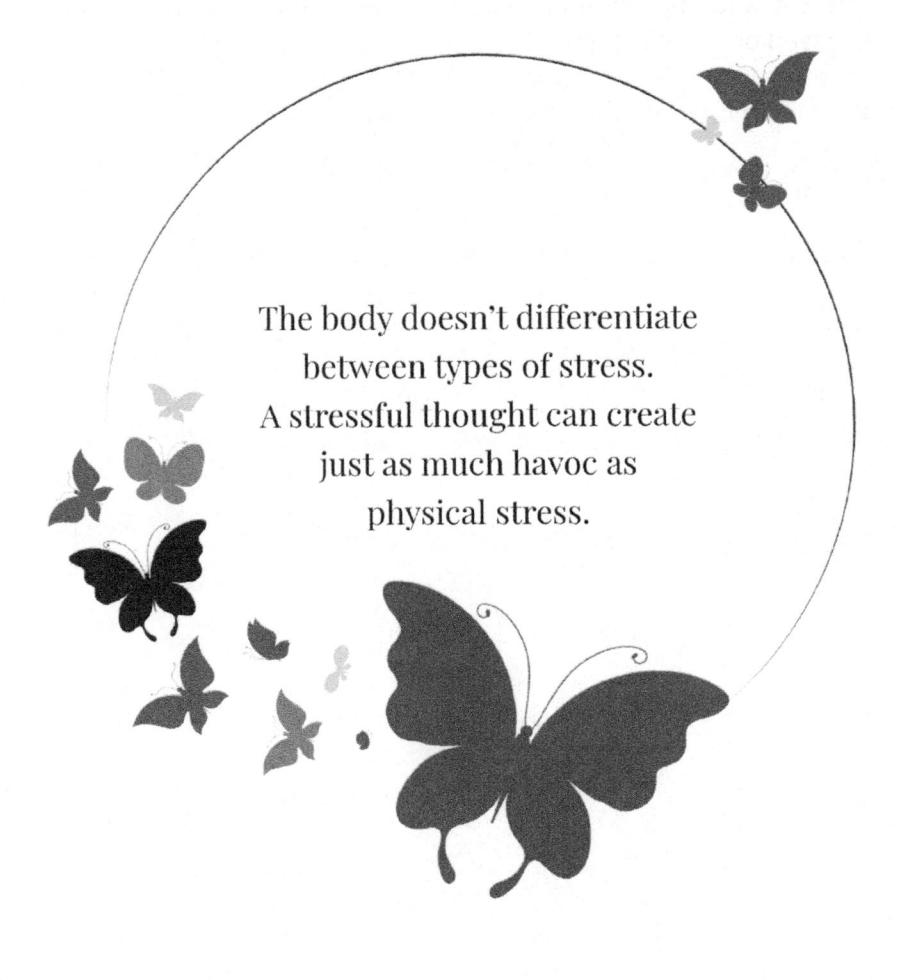

> The body doesn't differentiate between types of stress. A stressful thought can create just as much havoc as physical stress.

CHAPTER 16

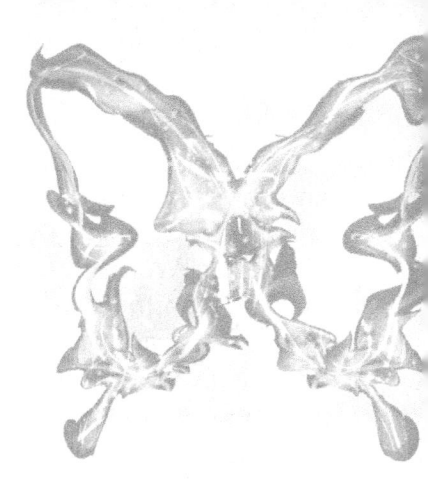

PHYSIOLOGY

Before venturing into this section, we want to reiterate that, in no way, is this an attempt to diagnose or give medical advice. It's information and education to help guide you in understanding what you really need to interpret the signals your body is giving you so you can address the root cause of the symptoms and heal rather than getting caught in a cycle of naming symptoms and suppressing them.

Diagnosis: Does It Even Matter?

The number of official diagnoses is absolutely frightening. There are over 69,000 ICD-10-CM diagnosis codes in the United States alone. (https://en.wikipedia.org/wiki/ICD-10)

Approximately 200 of those diagnoses are identified as autoimmune conditions, including heart disease and diabetes, but only about 20 solid tests are available for autoimmune diagnosis.

Studies show that about one in every seven people has a diagnosed autoimmune condition and that millions are unaware their symptoms are connected to an autoimmune disease.

An estimated 50 million Americans live with autoimmune diseases. There are 332 million people in America. That's about 15% of the population. Women are well known to have more powerful immune systems than men, which may produce more powerful autoimmune responses. Autoimmune diseases aren't always distinct, as multiple disorders can strike the same person simultaneously. Autoimmune diseases are among the ten leading causes of death among women up to the age of 65. Source: Autoimmune Association

Nearly half of all Americans suffer from at least one chronic disease including: cancer, diabetes, hypertension, stroke, heart disease, respiratory disease, arthritis, obesity, and oral diseases.
Source: https://www.ncbi.nlm.nih.gov/pmc/articles/PMC5876976/

You're probably reading this book because you (or your kids, spouse, parent, or best friend) are dealing with symptoms and struggling to figure out what's going on and how to get on a path to actual healing. Perhaps the doctors you've seen so far can't seem to find an "official diagnosis" or they can't give you a label for what you're experiencing, and the attempts you've made to correct the issues haven't worked.

No matter what's going on, please know... YOU ARE NOT CRAZY!

You might feel that way, as you've been dismissed by the medical community because they can't tie your symptoms up into a neat little diagnosis and, therefore, don't know how to help you. And you're tired of feeling the way you do and just want some answers, but you feel like you're going in circles.

Even if you don't have an official diagnosis or the doctors keep telling you that you are "normal," that *doesn't mean there's nothing wrong.*

As we discussed in the last chapter on labs, it may mean that the symptoms you are experiencing either aren't bad enough yet for the medical community to label it as a disease or condition, or it means that no one has been looking in the right places.

If you have been given a name to label what you are experiencing, but you feel like there's still more to the story because the medication or the support you are getting isn't helping you feel better, then you're probably right: something got missed.

To help recognize some red flags that may be waving right in front of you (and your doctors), below are a list of terms, names, and conditions we have found to be precursors to autoimmune, or they are full blown indicators that autoimmune is actually present but the practitioner you are working with isn't experienced enough with autoimmune to know that or to be alerted to look any further.

They are also all conditions that can be reversed (completely without medication) when their root causes are addressed.

Here are a list of common terms, names, and diagnoses people are given that may be indicators that autoimmune is hiding in the shadows or is already in effect:

- Hypothyroidism
- IBS or irritable bowel syndrome
- Chronic fatigue syndrome
- Any heart related condition
- Anxiety disorder
- Migraines
- Adrenal dysfunction or adrenal fatigue
- Hormone imbalance
- Chronic or post-partum depression
- Metabolic syndrome
- Reactive hypoglycemia
- Prediabetes
- Cystic acne
- Anaphylaxis (or serious allergies to foods or other substances)
- Hypersensitivity disease (this where people have reactions to things such as perfumes, chemicals, foods, light, sounds, textures, or materials.)
- Arthritis

- Inflammation
- Leaky gut/intestinal permeability
- Mast cell activation

Or your labs are indicating things such as:

- Autoimmune process indicators: Low triglycerides, high HDL with normal to high total cholesterol.
- TSH - High or Low
- Elevated antibodies such as TPO/TAA/ANA which indicate that your body is killing off cells faster than the body can create them.

Or (and this is our favorite "diagnosis") you might be told you have an "idiopathic condition" which means "a condition of unknown origin." Basically, the doctor is agreeing that you have something going on, but has no idea what it is. So, they give it a fancy name and maybe even prescribe some medication and send you on your way.

At least with the diagnosis of "idiopathic condition," you're being acknowledged for having something going on. What isn't okay, is when your complaints or symptoms are dismissed, and you don't feel validated or heard.

For example, when you see a practitioner about your symptoms and you're told:

- You're a new mom (or you have little kids at home) so it's normal to feel tired or out of balance or depressed.
- You are working too hard and just need to "relax," meditate, or do some yoga.
- You're experiencing menopausal symptoms and it's normal to feel awful.

So, you're dismissed with no answers on what you can do about what you're experiencing other than stop complaining, suck it up, and go away. And here's the thing; just because it's common for many people to experience something **does not** make it NORMAL or healthy.

Conventional and many functional medical doctors are trained to diagnose and prescribe. So, of course, that is the approach they take to solving patient complaints.

Interestingly, diagnosis isn't that important if you want to *address the underlying root causes* of the symptoms.

Understanding the message your body is trying to deliver with the symptoms is critical. Knowing why the body is behaving the way it is will bring far more benefit in the healing process than being able to call it by name.

If someone shows up at your front door, just because he introduces himself as John Doe doesn't mean you know why he's there, what he wants, or what it has to do with you. You have to ask questions, interpret the answers, and have a conversation with John to know what's going on. And even then, you still may not understand all you need to know.

If John doesn't speak the same language as you, even if you ask those questions and attempt to have that conversation, if you don't understand the words he's using to answer your questions or if he doesn't understand the language you're using to ask your questions, then you still won't know why he's there.

And if John is desperate enough to get you to understand, he might start yelling at you or getting upset. He may refuse to leave until you fix whatever problem he came to tell you about.

But again, no matter how loud he gets or how long he stays, if you can't understand what he's saying, you will still be confused. Maybe you will try to gently convince him to go away, or eventually you might threaten him to force him to leave because you're becoming alarmed by him and just want him to leave your property.

Even if John goes away temporarily because of your threats, if his message is important, he will return again and again trying to deliver that message.

At this point, you see John as a threat, but what if he's really there to help you because he knows something that could save your life, and that's what he's trying to tell you? If you shut him out, ignore him, or even call the police to take him away and do not get the information he's trying to deliver, you'll miss out on the message that will save your life.

Think of how this analogy can be applied to exactly what's going on in your health and your life right now. What signals is your body giving you every day in an attempt to communicate a message to you?

Your foggy brain, joint pain, bloating, or anxiety are pieces of information your body is lovingly using to communicate with you. Your body is your friend speaking a language you simply may not understand. Just because the message isn't clear to you (or to your doctor) doesn't mean the message (or the messenger) should be suppressed, ignored, or chased away.

Kirstin recently reflected on the day she finally got the diagnosis of celiac disease.

I was actually thrilled. I had been searching for answers for quite some time to my digestive issues, weight gain, fatigue, acne, hormone imbalances, and severe allergy episodes.

"Now," I thought, "I will finally get better."

I was told to stop eating gluten, was given some medication, a bunch of supplements, and an epi-pen for the allergy episodes and was sent on my merry way. As if, everything was now fixed.

And even though I did feel a little better after eliminating gluten from my diet, most of the symptoms remained. In other words, my body was trying to tell me that just because I had a name, that didn't mean that I actually understood.

The problem was: my body and I.... we weren't speaking the same language. I needed to learn how to interpret the symptoms and the communication my body was using to tell me what it needed, what was going on, and what I could do to fix it.

Essentially, the body was saying: "Hey I'm out of balance, and I need help." And this imbalance could stem from emotional, mental, and/or physical symptoms, but all three are connected at all times. So, when you impact one, you impact the others.

For example: If you are worried about a math test (which is an emotional response), because you think you aren't smart (which is a mental response), you may experience stomach pains and diarrhea (which is obviously a physical response.)

That physical response may then begin to happen any time you sense any worry or feel dumb, and will continue to cause damage and potentially create an even bigger set of problems.

If you simply treat the symptom of diarrhea and see it only as a physical problem and don't get to the root cause of that problem (thinking you aren't smart) then, at best, you will only suppress that symptom and it will show up in another way in an attempt to communicate that there's an underlying problem not being addressed.

Everything in your system is connected all the time. At no time are you only experiencing something emotionally and not physically and mentally or having a physical symptom that's not connected to a mental and emotional response.

They are all influencing and impacting each other, **always**.

Chapter Takeaways

- We are a country that is hung up on labels (diagnosis) and the name isn't the cause. It's just a name for a collection of symptoms. The root cause is more important to healing than the diagnosis.

- One in seven people in the Unites States has been diagnosed with an autoimmune disease and millions are walking around undiagnosed.

- Your symptoms are not "all in your head." You are not crazy. If you are feeling dismissed, find another practitioner who understands how to help you find the root cause and get you on the path to transformational health

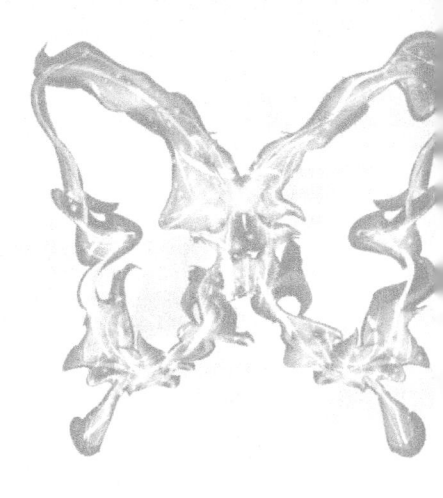

CHAPTER 17

MEDICATION

With the support of their prescribing doctor, most of our clients wean off their medications while we help them identify and dissolve the root causes of their symptoms.

Medications have their place, but most (Americans especially) are unnecessarily or over medicated. The average American takes four prescription medications, and many are taking the medication for longer than the medication was designed to be taken.

Proton Pump Inhibitors (PPIs) for example, are generally recommended to be taken for two to eight weeks. PPIs are supposed to help with GERD and acid reflux by reducing the amount of stomach acid produced, which then causes its own side effects. Make no mistake, literally EVERY medication has side or direct effects because they block pathways and circumvent the body's natural functionality.

Let's continue to use PPIs as an example to explain this cascade of side effects further. The most common side effects for PPIs include constipation, headache, diarrhea, and vomiting. Some of the most serious PPI side effects involve a range of kidney problems including kidney failure and end-stage renal disease. Because PPIs directly shut down proton pumps in the body, it makes the kidney related side effects a double whammy because reduction in protons cause a reduction in potassium which causes a reduction in hydrochloric acid (HCL) which is a key component of a healthy functioning immune system. Potassium also helps to stabilize the pH of the blood to remain alkaline, which is also incredibly important to staying healthy. So the irony is that most people who have GERD or acid reflux have it because of a lack of stomach acid, not too much stomach acid. Which means, taking PPIs makes the low stomach acid problem worse, suppresses the immune system, causes acidity in the blood pH, puts unnecessary stress on the kidneys, and puts a strain on the entire body causing long term problems and damage. But PPIs are one of the most commonly doctor prescribed (and over the counter) medications on the market today. One pharmaceutical company reported PPI sales of $72.5 billion between 1992 and 2017. Bonkers, right?

> **PPIs suppress the immune system, which means they lower your natural ability to fight disease and heal.**

Thyroid medication is another great example of where there is a likely chance of over (or unnecessary) medicating. When the TSH (Thyroid Stimulating Hormone) marker is not in "normal range" it is our recommendation to run a full thyroid panel, including antibodies, to get a better overall picture of thyroid function so you can understand where the break down is occurring.

- Is it because the immune system is attacking the thyroid?
- Is there a thyroid hormone conversion problem?
- Is it a challenge with the production of thyroid hormone?

Most doctors only focus on the basic marker of TSH. Ironically even though TSH is a thyroid marker, it isn't actually produced by the thyroid. Most practitioners (including endocrinologists who are supposed to be experts in hormones, thyroid, and the entire endocrine system) don't bother to run thyroid antibodies to determine if the problem is due to Hashimoto's (immune system attack) because even if the antibodies come back elevated, it won't change their treatment plan. In most cases, you'll still receive a prescription for thyroid medication and be sent on your way, which won't solve the underlying reason for the thyroid issue. Simply medicating, and not correcting the root cause typically causes more health problems later on.

Let's look at why.

Assuming you have a thyroid and it hasn't been removed for some reason, how does taking thyroid medication directly improve thyroid function? If you have hypothyroid (underactive thyroid), how does taking thyroid medication help the thyroid produce optimal amounts of its own hormone? It doesn't.

Since the hormone is being taken exogenously, the thyroid has no reason to produce optimal amounts of hormone. And the patient now has to perform a juggling act, constantly adjusting their medication to get their TSH marker in a specific range instead of supporting the thyroid naturally with the right nutrients responsible for proper thyroid physiology along with lifestyle, energetic, and emotional pieces needed for thyroid health. And as we'll discuss later in the book, one of the best things you can do to support your thyroid is to express yourself to your satisfaction. In other words, communicate effectively. When was the last time your doctor put down the prescription pad and recommended speaking your mind to help balance your thyroid and increase functionality?

There's a new commercial for a pharmaceutical that treats a condition called EPI (exocrine pancreatic insufficiency). It's marketed to people whose pancreas is not producing enough enzymes to break down food properly and absorb nutrients. It contains lipase which breaks down fats, protease which breaks down proteins, and amylase which breaks down carbohydrates (sugars). According to the commercial, people with the following symptoms are candidates: cystic fibrosis, chronic inflammation of the pancreas, or blockage of the pancreatic ducts.

Then the most common side effects are mentioned. Stomach (abdominal) pain, bloating, trouble passing stool, nausea, vomiting, diarrhea, worsening of painful swollen joints (gout), or allergic reactions, including trouble with breathing, skin rashes, or swollen lips. This drug may also increase your chance of having a bowel disorder called fibrosing colonopathy. This is absurd. Why not simply take an over-the-counter plant-based digestive enzyme supplement containing lipase, protease, and amylase without the drug related side effects? On the website for the drug, it even says: "Pancreatic enzyme replacement therapies (PERTs) are the standard of care for EPI." A plant-based digestive enzyme qualifies as pancreatic enzyme replacement therapy.

In addition to the side effects, and unnecessary prescribing, systematic reviews of hospital charts found that even properly prescribed drugs (aside from mis-prescribing, overdosing, or self-prescribing) cause about 1.9 million hospitalizations a year. Another 840,000 hospitalized patients are given drugs that cause serious adverse reactions for a total of 2.74 million serious adverse drug reactions. About 128,000 people die from drugs prescribed to them. This makes prescription drugs a major health risk, ranking 4th with stroke as a leading cause of death.[1]

HACK:

If the name of the drug is not mentioned on an advertisement, the pharmaceutical company does not have to list the side effects of the drug.

One of our mentors calls them *harma*ceuticals.

Certain medication can also deplete nutrients. See the next page for a list of nutrients that some common medications deplete:

Drug Induced Nutrient Depletion

Medication Type	Common Names	Depleted Vitamins	Depleted Minerals	Other
Blood Pressure	Atacand		Zinc, Magnesium, Calcium, Phosphorus	CoQ10
	Lisinopril		Zinc	
	Beta Blocker			CoQ10, Melatonin
Cholesterol	Lipitor, Zocor			CoQ10
	Questran, Colestipol	A, Folic Acid, B12, D, E, K	Iron	
	Lopid	E		CoQ10
Diabetes	Metformin, Glimepiride	Folic Acid, B12		CoQ10
Pain Anti-inflammatory	NSAID – Ibuprofen, Advil, Motrin	Folic Acid	Zinc, Iron	Melatonin
	Aspirin	B3, B6, Folic Acid, B9, C, D	Zinc, Calcium, Potassium, Iron	
	Corticosteroid – Prednisone, hydrocortisone	A, B6, Folic Acid, B12, C, D	Zinc, Magnesium, Calcium, Potassium, Selenium	DHEA, Protein, AA, Melatonin
Heartburn/Reflux	Zantac, Pepcid AC	B1, B2, B5, Biotin, Folic Acid, B12	Zinc, Magnesium	

	Prilosec	B1	Magnesium, Calcium, Phosphorus	
Hormone Replacement	Estrogen	B1, B2, B5, Biotin, Folic Acid, B12	Zinc, Magnesium	
Oral Contraceptive		A, B1, B5, B6, Biotin, Folic Acid, B12, C	Zinc, Magnesium	
Birth Control		B2, B6, Biotin	Magnesium	
Antidepressants	Zoloft, Prozac	B1, Biotin	Magnesium, Calcium	CoQ10

Source: https://www.doctorsbeyondmedicine.com/listing/drug-induced-nutrient-depletion

Bruce Ames, a biochemist at the University of California, Berkeley is convinced the standard high-calorie, low-nutrient diet is responsible for many chronic diseases, including cancer. Ames has found that even subtle micronutrient deficiencies, far below the levels to produce acute deficiency diseases, can cause damage to DNA that may lead to cancer. Studying cultured human cells, he has found that deficiencies of vitamin C, E, B12, B6, niacin, folic acid, iron, or zinc appears to mimic radiation by causing single and double strand DNA breaks, oxidative lesions, or both. Precursors to cancer.[2] And medications may be the reason for these nutrient deficiencies.

Chapter Takeaways

- The United States is the sickest first world country and autoimmune disease and chronic illness are increasing at an alarming rate.

- Your symptoms are not all in your head.

- Treating symptoms is not the answer.

- All medications have side effects.

- Medications can deplete nutrients.

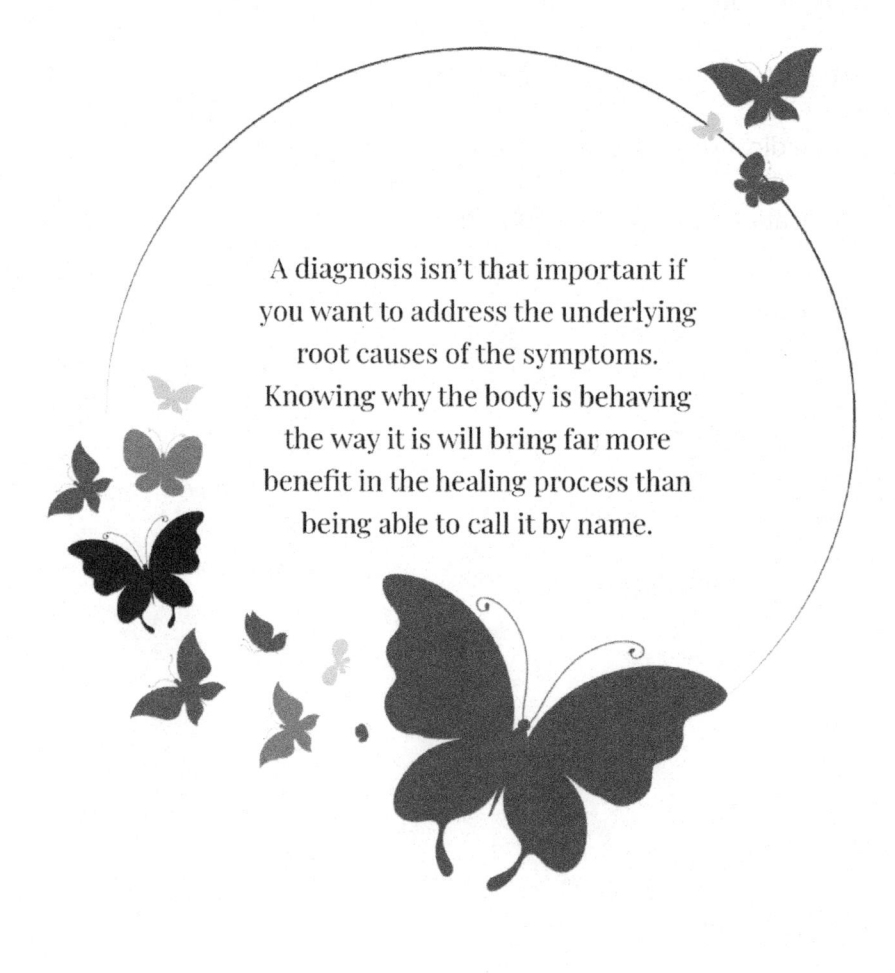

A diagnosis isn't that important if you want to address the underlying root causes of the symptoms. Knowing why the body is behaving the way it is will bring far more benefit in the healing process than being able to call it by name.

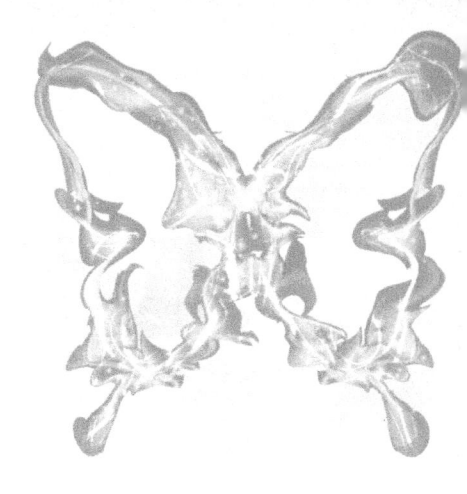

CHAPTER 18

EPIGENETICS

Earlier, we covered the fight-or-flight response, the rest-and-digest response, and how the adrenals play a role in the hormones created during the sympathetic response. We also talked about how there's an enormous difference between being in fight-or-flight, some of the time versus all of the time.

Now, we will go deeper and show you how those same chemicals and hormones impact you on a genetic level through epigenetics. Epigenetics is what "does the business" so-to-speak, and we'll do our best to communicate how important this is and how it all works.

Epigenetics is a relatively new science that has to do with genes as the name suggests. Every cell in our body, except red blood cells, contains genes. Up until recently, it was thought that the genes control the cells, but we now know that's not true. Dr. Bruce Lipton discusses an experiment in his book *The Biology of Belief* where he plucked the nucleus out of the cell where the genes are held, and the cell carried on with completely normal behavior. It didn't change the behavior of the cell at all even though it was missing its nucleus.

Let's discuss exactly what that means and why it's important to understand if you want transformational healing.

Every cell, with the exception of red blood cells, contains a nucleus. If you look inside the nucleus, you'll find chromosomes. Men have XY chromosomes; women have XX chromosomes. Each chromosome is made up of DNA tightly coiled many times around proteins called histones that support its structure. The end of chromosomes are called telomeres, which play a central role in aging. A section of DNA is a gene. To keep it really simple, genes are the blueprints to create proteins.

Your body is a protein-creating machine, and proteins are the building blocks of every part of your body. Your skin has proteins in it called collagen and elastin. Muscles have proteins called actin and myosin. Enzymes like lipase, protease, and amylase are proteins. Even antibodies are proteins. So, we need proper nutrition to give our body the various amino acids so it can synthesize or produce proteins that make different components that form and maintain your body. An example of how this process works is this: Proteins make cells and cells make up tissues. Tissues make organs or glands, which makes up systems. Systems make up our whole body.

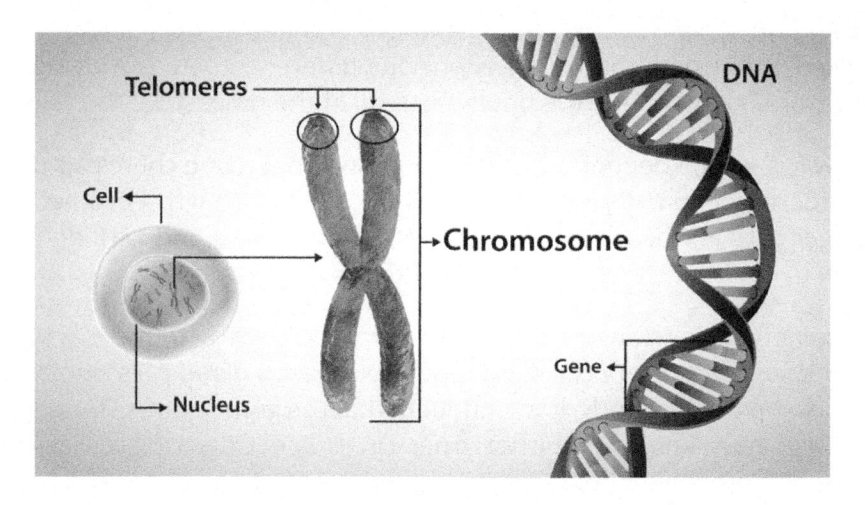

Here's a riddle for you:

You're stranded on a desert island and your only food options are bananas, sprouts, peaches, chocolate, or kale. Which food option will keep you alive for an extended period of time? Believe it or not, it's the chocolate because we cannot live without fat and protein. We can live without carbohydrates however, and the chocolate contains the protein and fat needed to survive.

There's a metabolic process called gluconeogenesis where the body can convert protein and fat into glucose. This is why you do not need to consume glucose to live and why consuming protein and fat is critical. We're not suggesting you don't eat carbohydrates or eat only chocolate, we're highlighting just how truly amazing the body is, as it's the greatest instrument you'll ever own.

The word epigenetics translates to mean "above the genes." Earlier, we talked a little bit about how your feelings and emotions create chemistry in the body. Let's expand upon that and discuss how feelings and emotions influence gene expression, which ultimately determines whether you are on the poor health trajectory or the ideal health trajectory.

Epigenetics - Above the Genes

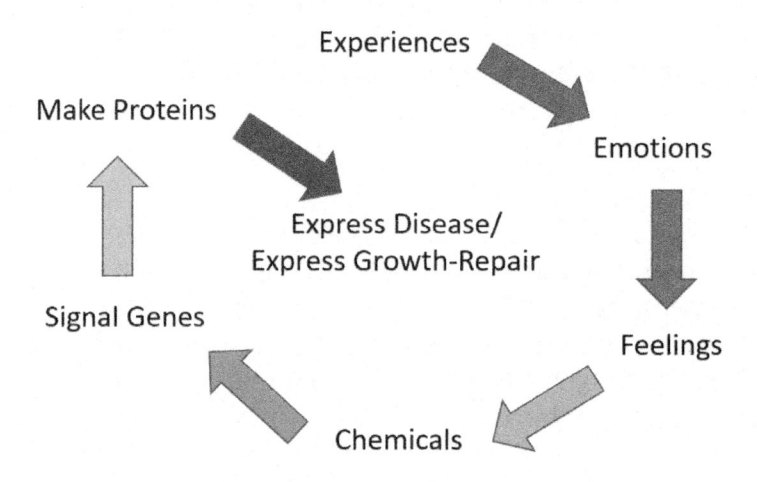

```
              Experiences
                   ↘
Make Proteins              Emotions
     ↑         Express Disease/
               Express Growth-Repair
                                ↓
Signal Genes                Feelings
         ↖                ↙
              Chemicals
```

Experiences in our environment create emotions like fear, anger, pride, and happiness. Those emotions create feelings like excitement, annoyance, purposefulness, and gratitude. Each feeling produces a chemical (hormone or neuropeptide) that corresponds to that feeling. Some examples are as follows: oxytocin is the love and bonding hormone. Serotonin is the feel-good hormone, which eventually converts into melatonin, which helps us sleep. Cortisol and adrenaline are both produced by the adrenal glands when we're in fight-or-flight mode. Feelings produce chemicals and those chemicals signal genes to make proteins.

Over 140,000 different proteins make up the body and proteins create structure and function. There's actually a gene that makes proteins specifically to suppress tumors. But energy draining emotions and feelings can actually suppress (or downregulate) genes that make that tumor-suppressing protein, making the body more vulnerable to tumor growth.

Chapter 18 - Epigenetics | 111

Our feelings and emotions can either cause genes to express or be silent. And the proteins that are made determine whether we express disease or growth/repair.

We can also look at it backwards. Disease or growth/repair is determined by proteins, which are determined by the genes that are signaled, which are determined by what chemicals our body produces, which are determined by our feelings, emotions, and experiences.

These gene expressions, triggered by feelings, emotions, and experiences have been scientifically proven to be passed down from generation to generation.

In a study conducted by Brian Diaz and Kerry Ressler at Emory University, published in *Nature Neuroscience*, generational fear was shown passing from one mouse generation to the next. In the experiment, mouse parents were exposed to electrical shocks whenever they smelled the scent of cherry blossom and almond. Subsequently, when the children and grandchildren of the mice smelled the scent of cherry blossom, they became startled even though they had never been exposed to the scent or shocked before the experiment. It was also discovered that the offspring of the shocked mouse parents also had more neurons that detected the cherry blossom scent than mice whose parents hadn't been shocked when exposed to that scent. Such fear can be transmitted at the level of the DNA: Researchers found that the DNA in the sperm cells was imprinted with the association between fear and the scent of cherry blossom. A gene that codes for the molecule that detects this odor carried a chemical marker that they postulated may have changed the behavior of the gene.[1]

> Gene expression ultimately determines whether you are on the poor health trajectory or the ideal health trajectory, and is influenced by thoughts, feelings, and emotions.

The ability to inherit a fear or trauma response from your parents may have developed as a survival instinct to learn what can threaten your life without having to be exposed directly to the threat. In modern society however, this biological adaptation has a dark side that may explain how seemingly irrational phobias, anxiety, and posttraumatic stress disorder develop-to say nothing of your everyday fears, such as fear of never having enough money or fear of being rejected by those you love.[2]

What's important about this study is how it sheds light on why you may be experiencing the specific fears, feelings, and emotions you have regularly, especially if you notice similar emotional threads throughout your family. Do you notice similar repeating traumas in your family like generational abuse? This is incredibly common and epigenetics may be responsible as part of the "learning" that occurs from one generation to the next through gene expression.

Since trauma is often hidden and not talked about because of fear and shame, many people don't realize the trauma has been experienced by many in the generations before them. When we work with clients, we often discover that traumas, such as sexual abuse, follow family blood lines many generations deep. The combination of the trauma being passed down genetically because of epigenetics while also staying hidden because that trauma has been kept a secret has made the trauma response more powerful over time. This is why it's common to also see shame related symptoms such as anxiety, depression, heart disease, celiac disease, IBS, Crohn's, ulcerative colitis, and stomach, ovarian, uterine, and breast cancers thread through families with a history of similar abuse.

The negative emotional impact of this type of abuse often presents as physical symptoms appearing in the gut, sexual organs, and heart as they are energetically the areas of the body that tend to hold unprocessed shame, our identity and sense of "Self," and our ability to accept love and love Self.

This is why it is incredibly helpful in the healing process to not only surface, express, and learn how to properly process your personal responses to trauma, but to also get a glimpse into your connection to your past and the experiences of the people in the generations before you. Understanding the threads and connections can help break generational trauma and free not only yourself, but everyone else in the bloodline.

We are going to delve much deeper in the Soul Section of this book into how experiences can create trauma responses, which can result in symptoms and disease, so you get a clear understanding of what you need to get to the root of what's causing your negative health trajectory and what you need for transformational health.

Thoughts Control Your Chemistry

Ninety percent of the thoughts you have today are the same thoughts that you had yesterday. If you keep having the same thoughts and repeating the same patterns every day, then you're not going to trigger new genes and new ways, and your tomorrow is going to pretty much be the same as your today.

The "Feeling Thinking Loop" explained by Dr. Joe Dispenza in *Becoming Supernatural: How Common People Are Doing the Uncommon,* looks like this: When you have a thought, that thought creates chemicals to make your feelings match what you're thinking. Those feelings then lead to more thoughts.

For example, let's say you have thoughts about being overwhelmed. The body produces chemicals, so you physically and emotionally feel the overwhelm. Then those feelings lead to more overwhelming thoughts. That triggers the body to produce more chemicals that make you more overwhelmed, and those overwhelming feelings create more overwhelming thoughts. Now you are caught in the Feeling Thinking Loop. Your thoughts are driving your feelings and your feelings are driving your thoughts.

Or maybe you're at work one day and your boss sends you an e-mail with the subject line: "Come into my office when you get in." You think, *What did I do wrong?* And then that thought produces chemicals which lead you to feel like you've done something wrong, which lead to more thoughts connected to things you could have done wrong. *Did I miss a deadline? Is there some kind of a problem?* Then off you go....

If we start our day thinking about our problems, we will tap into the memories associated with those problems. This connection between the memories and the problems creates recognized feelings and emotions like sadness, worry, regret, and grief that drive our thoughts. If we cannot think differently than how we feel, the past drives our feelings and actions, and therefore, our past will become our future. So inevitably, the choices we made yesterday are going to be the same choices we make tomorrow, and we are going to keep repeating the same patterns, and our life, heath, and circumstance will stay the same.

Points to Ponder

- Every thought you think produces corresponding internal chemistry. In other words, the body reacts in kind. Emotions aren't good or bad (though you might like some more than others), they are all a necessary part of the human experience. When we are out of balance and chronically dwelling on (or trying to suppress) thoughts like fear, anger, and worry, the body will create chemistry that will influence genes and lead to disease.

- We use less than 2% of our DNA. The remaining 98% science actually calls junk DNA. Nature works off the "use it or lose it" principle. So, over thousands of years, if it hasn't evolved away, then what's it really doing there? Science is starting to discover that the "unused" DNA isn't junk and that it is useful and plays a role in epigenetics.

- Earlier, in Chapter 13: Adrenal Function, we explained when we feel safe, those feelings release a flood of 1,400 biochemical changes that promote growth and repair. When we feel anger, hurt, stress, jealousy, rage, competition, or frustration, which are all connected to feeling unsafe, it releases about 1,200 chemicals into the body creating a negative gene expression.

Research done by Keiko Hayashi PhD, found that diabetics, after watching a one-hour-long comedy program, had 39 genes upregulated (turned on or activated). Fourteen of those genes were related to natural killer cell activity (a part of the immune system's innate ability to control tumor growth and stop the spread of microbial infections).

Interestingly, killer cell activity has nothing to do with glucose regulation, but the patient's glucose was better controlled after watching the comedy routine than after listening to a diabetes health lecture on a completely different day.[3] So, laughing is pretty powerful stuff too.

DNA is composed of two layers. One layer is old, evolved from millions of years of evolution. It's fixed and very hard to change. The other layer is the epigenetic layer, which is dynamic and interactive.

Here's an example of how the physical environment influences gene expression through the dynamic and interactive layer.

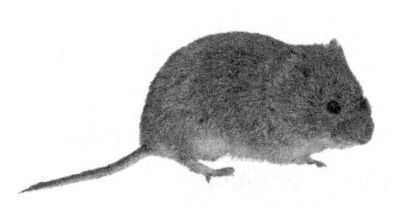

This is a picture of a rodent known as a vole which are born with one gene that determines a thick coat, and another gene that determines a thin coat. If they're born in the summer, the thin gene turns on. If they're born in the winter, the thick coat gene turns on. The gene expression is determined by the environment they're born into. Crocodiles have the gene for both sexes, and the temperature of the environment that they're born into determines which gender they end up being.

Here's how the emotional environment impacts gene expression.

All energy has a frequency and all frequencies carry information. When we change our frequency, we change our energy.

Energy *draining* emotions like anger, fear, resentment, judgement, shame, and guilt have a low frequency. The lower the frequency, the more heavy or dense the body feels, lowering its ability to heal or stay healthy.

Energy *raising* emotions like love, gratitude, inspiration, and joy have a much higher frequency. The higher or faster the frequency of emotions we have, the freer and lighter the body feels, which shifts the body away from disease and towards health.

Energy draining emotions are often created by an underlying perceived trauma triggered by an event with a high emotional charge that left you (or one of your ancestors) in shame, fear, or pain, and branded into your biology. This then caused the genes that were activated to keep you stuck on a poor health trajectory. Why? Because the environment influences gene expression, genes create proteins, and it's the proteins that express disease or express growth/repair.

In order to change that gene expression, the energy draining emotional pattern connected to the past trauma must be rewired to a higher frequency emotion. Altering the emotional connection (environment) will allow the healthy genes to be expressed and the genes for disease to be silenced.

Chapter Takeaways

- You are not destined to your genes because your parents or grandparents had a particular disease or condition.

- Experiences create emotions. Emotions create feelings. Feelings create chemistry. Chemistry signals genes to upregulate or downregulate. Genes that are expressed (upregulated) create proteins. These proteins determine health or disease.

- Symptoms and disease are influenced by generational trauma and will appear in areas of the body that correspond with the emotion connected with that trauma. This is why you will often see specific types of abuse commonly presenting as similar physical symptoms.

PART 4

SOUL

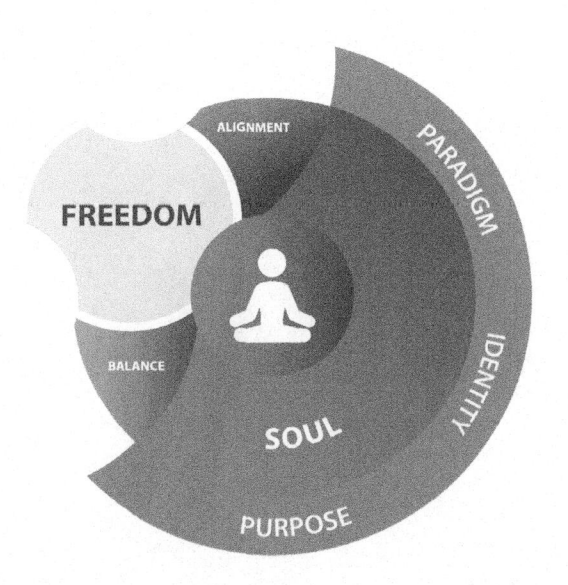

N ow you understand more about the science, genetics, and physiology behind the healing process, you should also have more tangible information on what you may need for long-term health, happiness, and fulfillment. The studies and details reviewed so far should also have given you more insight into why healing is more than just breathing and "letting go of stress."

In this Soul Section, we're going to take a deep dive into how your purpose, identity, and paradigm influence your entire system emotionally, mentally, and physically, so that you can recognize and remove the blocks that put you on the destructive health trajectory you are currently on and flip you on to the path to transformational health.

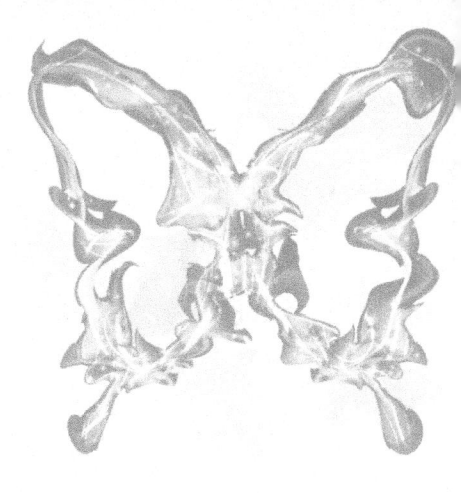

CHAPTER 19

THE FRACTURED SOUL

When you feel stuck, splintered, unfulfilled, or disconnected emotionally, the body reacts as if it's in real physical danger.

For many years, we've worked with clients who have autoimmune disease, chronic stress, thyroid dysfunction, hormone imbalance, and related issues and found patterns that cause the body to go into "attack mode" and destroy its own healthy cells and tissues.

One of these reasons has to do with what we call a "fractured soul."

When we use the term "soul" what we mean is "the essence of you." It's the part that you can't measure or touch, but you know it's there. It's the part that makes you… **you.**

It's your:

- Thoughts
- Feelings
- Beliefs
- Values
- Identity
- Perspective

- Personality
- Purpose
- Paradigm
- Spirit

The soul is one of the three crucial components of healing, along with the nutrition and science, and is typically the most overlooked piece in the healing journey.

People so often tell us, "I want to get back to being ME!"

This usually means, that their soul is "fractured."

Their identity, thoughts, beliefs, and purpose have been squashed and shifted in a way that they no longer even recognize themselves at a core level, and they no longer feel "whole." This causes a splintering of Self, which can show up as symptoms such as digestive distress, anxiety, fatigue, pain, weight gain, foggy-brain, hormone imbalance, and disease.

An incredibly common reason why the body and soul become disconnected and splintered is due to underlying and unaddressed low frequency issues stemming from fear, shame, trauma, or other emotional distress as discussed in the last chapter on epigenetics. These low frequencies can become subconsciously anchored into identity, belief, and value at a core level in an effort to protect you from danger.

This hardwiring to "stay safe" can be helpful so we don't wander off of high buildings or put our hands directly onto a hot stove, but it can also be restrictive and even destructive when the need to "stay safe" overrides our dreams, desires, and optimal health.

When the soul continues to stay splintered, and vibrate at a low frequency, it's nearly impossible to get on the ideal healing trajectory without a custom strategy that includes a process to bring the splintered pieces back together by addressing underlying emotional root causes.

Chapter Takeaways

- A fractured soul is when you are disconnected from how you feel due to trauma or underlying belief systems that are trying to keep you safe but are really causing you to miss the underlying message the body is attempting to deliver to you about what is wrong and what it needs to heal.

- When the soul is fractured, it often presents as physical symptoms such as digestive distress, anxiety, hormone imbalance, fatigue, pain, and disease.

- Unaddressed fear, shame, trauma, or other emotional distress is often anchored to core identity, and our hardwired need to stay safe can override dreams, desires, and optimal health.

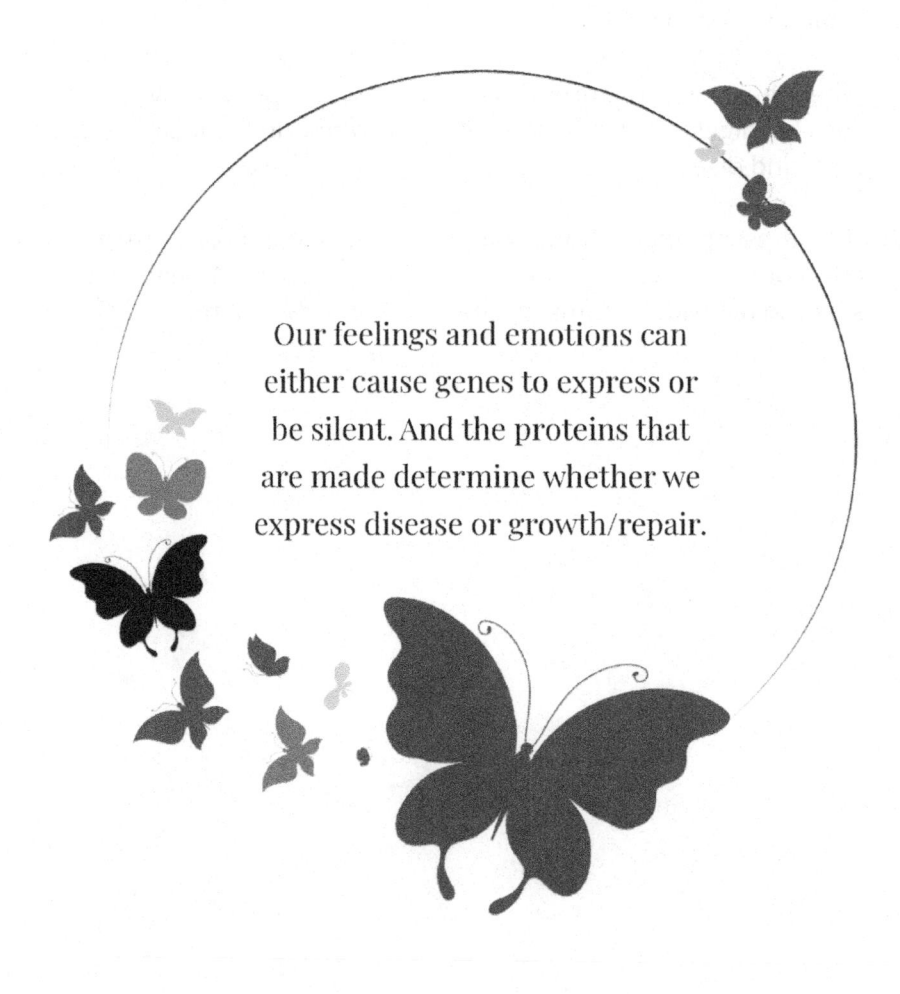

Our feelings and emotions can either cause genes to express or be silent. And the proteins that are made determine whether we express disease or growth/repair.

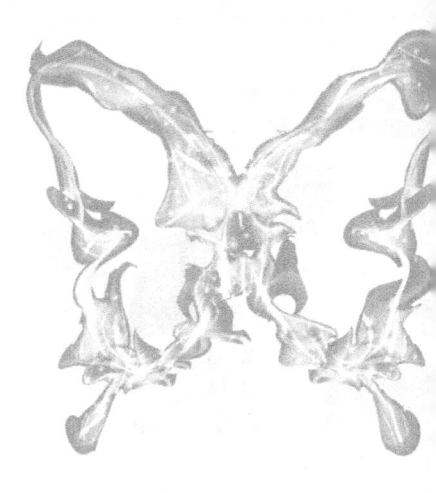

CHAPTER 20

WHAT'S YOUR PURPOSE?

Do you feel you were meant for something more or different than the life experience you are having? Is there a disconnected feeling between your purpose and your life?

Purpose is a driving force and it's also a magnet. When you are clearly aware of your purpose, you can leverage the power of that driving force and obtain more of what you want in life. Clarity of purpose will also bring you a better understanding of why you specifically attract things (positive and negative) into your life. That awareness will empower you to alter your life, raise the vibration of energy in your body, and attract more joy, success, and the healthy life experience you desire.

When you are *unaware* of your purpose, or have a lack of clarity around it, you will still be driven in a direction but with no influence on the direction, and you will attract things into your life that typically lead to unhappiness, struggle, frustration, and ill health.

Your purpose is your raison d'être. It's the point of *everything*. You have a purpose even if you aren't consciously aware of what that purpose is. It's critical to shed light on your purpose because it's the power behind everything in your life.

When you are disconnected from purpose, it's difficult to understand yourself, your life, and the messages all around you.

When you are sick or fighting against chronic pain, stress, or fatigue, it can be difficult to see anything besides the symptoms. Your core purpose becomes eclipsed by finding a solution to your daily challenges.

When you are lost or disconnected from your sense of purpose, your body will resonate at a lower frequency and respond in fear because of the lack of direction. It needs an understanding of where you are going in order to feel safe. Purpose is what drives your decisions and actions. It's what makes you who you are.

That's why when you feel overwhelmed, lost, or depressed, it's difficult to understand what to do to feel better emotionally, mentally, or physically. Purpose is the driving force directly connected to the essence of who you are. When you lose that connection, the body becomes confused. It doesn't know how to support you, loses its sense of joy, and becomes lethargic and afraid.

If there's no sense of purpose, there's no sense of Self. If there's no sense of Self, the body doesn't recognize you. When you aren't recognized, the body becomes confused and scared, mistaking you as a threat. Which is often a trigger for an autoimmune attack, anxiety, depression, and illness.

Take a moment now and ask yourself:

- What's my purpose?
- Who am I?
- What are my top three life goals?
- What's my specific vision of my future?
- What is driving that vision?

If you are feeling stuck by these questions, don't panic. The good news is there is an answer for every one of them. You simply have lost your connection to those answers. Through the rest of the Soul Section, we are going to discuss not only the reason for that disconnection but also what you can do to reconnect and find your Self again.

My Purpose - Kirstin

My purpose is to continue to learn and grow personally and professionally so I can help others leverage their inherent ability to heal and live fulfilling, joy-filled lives. I know with certainty that every experience I've had to this point has led me directly toward that purpose, because I learned how to recognize my purpose and connect with it fully.

This is why I gravitate to people who are connected to their core purpose. Anthony and I spend tens of thousands of dollars every year upgrading our knowledge through books, workshops, courses, summits, events, business mentoring, and mindset coaching. It's why we each spend hundreds of hours working directly with clients, collaborating with other healing experts in various modalities, and connecting with our core Selves so we can teach others how to achieve true healing faster and more simply. I aim to be the embodiment of what healing is and actively live a transformational healing life.

My connection to that purpose drives me beyond the challenges that appear along the journey. Because, do not be mistaken, on the road to your purpose, you will absolutely be challenged, though it should never feel like suffering. Challenge is a necessary part of the growth, learning, and healing process. It's why I often "work" 70-hour weeks but don't feel wrecked by them. I know the challenge will be there, but don't get thrown off course by them. When we feel connected to purpose and know it's exactly what we were meant to do, the challenges will motivate you more. When you are unsure, feel like you are suffering, or have underlying hidden blocks, you will drop into a lower energy frequency of fear which will scare you, stop you, and often force you away from your purpose.

We have the most amazing team here at Nourish, because everyone on the team is connected with their purpose and is interested in learning and growing personally and professionally every day. They know that challenge is part of the process, though suffering is not, and the challenge is there to help them grow and reach even further. Each understands how their personal purpose supports the larger purpose of the company. And this compilation of purpose-driven people, moving toward a larger core mission is one of the reasons why our clients are so successful in reaching their health and life goals.

Here's an example of how when you are focused on purpose and the vision of your goals, you will not be stopped even if doubt or challenge creeps in.

Jennifer's Story

During one of our client coaching clinics, Jennifer, a woman who had just completed our yearlong *Health Freedom Program* popped onto the Zoom call. When we first met her, she was struggling with extreme fatigue, skin rashes, swollen eyes, brain fog, weight gain, headaches, lower back pain, and she had been diagnosed with MS and Lyme disease.

"I'm celebrating having more energy to do stuff around the house and am more mentally motivated. Last week I was super excited to quit my job, focus on my healing, and spend the summer with my kids before I start my new business. I was so excited! But when I went to resign I had so much anxiety, I couldn't do it. My symptoms started to come back, and I was feeling exhausted.

"Now that I've seen the vision of my own business and imagined what my life possibility holds, I hate my job even more. I started to see roadblocks getting in the way of that vision and started to question if I'm making the right decision. I felt paralyzed. Like I was in a holding pattern.

"But after doing the exercise on purpose you gave me, I realized what the block was. I couldn't see very far into the future before I started in this program because I didn't think I would live that long. Now I am feeling so much better, I'm thinking about the future and seeing farther than I ever have before.

"Before, I used to think, *Oh I'm just so thankful, given how sick I am, that I have a job that pays well so I can take care of my kids*. Now I have a vision that I can live past my 60s, I'm asking myself, '*Why am I in this job that I don't want to be in?*'

"I can have a life exactly how I want because I can see it and know I'm going to be alive for it! And if I'm alive for it, I better fully live it!"

Now that Jennifer could connect with herself and see a future, her purpose became clear. Her purpose was bigger than just trying to survive, it was about truly living, serving others with her new business, and leveraging every moment.

If you are living small and trying to "stay safe" because you can't see beyond your symptoms, it is likely you are struggling with your connection with your purpose.

Chapter Takeaways

- Your connection to your core purpose will drive your life and impact your health. When you feel disconnected or conflicted with your purpose, you are more likely to attract poor health and other challenges that do not make you feel safe.

- Feelings of overwhelm, depression, and discontent are signs that you are disconnected to the essence of who you are and why you exist, causing feelings of confusion and fear within your body.

- When you have no sense of purpose, you have no sense of Self, which can trigger an autoimmune attack and illness.

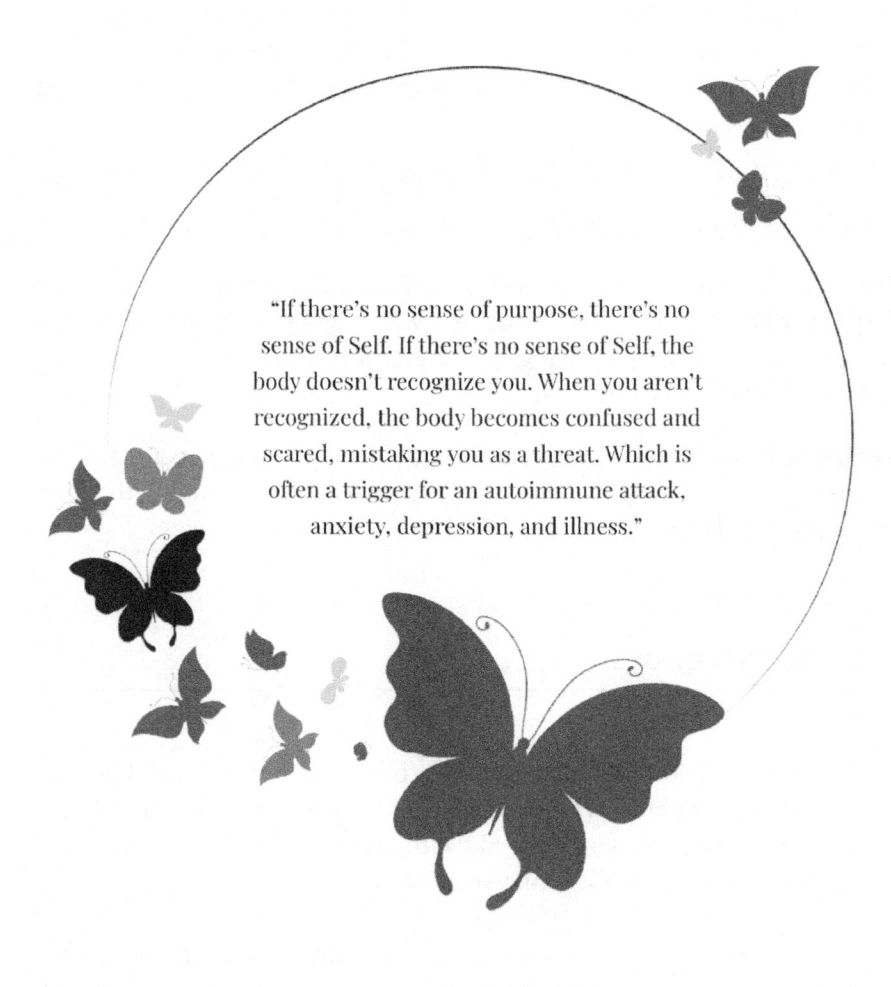

"If there's no sense of purpose, there's no sense of Self. If there's no sense of Self, the body doesn't recognize you. When you aren't recognized, the body becomes confused and scared, mistaking you as a threat. Which is often a trigger for an autoimmune attack, anxiety, depression, and illness."

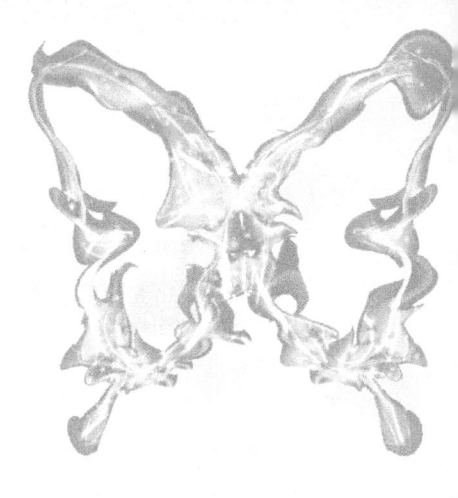

CHAPTER 21

IDENTITY

Identity is a powerful underlying driver controlling your life and everything in it. Every choice you make and every action you take are based on who you believe you are or who you were conditioned to think you were supposed to be.

Your subconscious identity is what drives your actions and beliefs, and it's based on your perception of what keeps you safe.

The subconscious spends a lot of effort searching for evidence to support and defend identity, even if that identity is ultimately working against what you say you want.

The belief of who you are (or who you think you are supposed to be), will also impact your:

- Symptoms
- Purpose
- Relationships
- Choices
- Perceptions
- Actions

- Health trajectory
- Life experience

Your identity drives choices, decisions, and health trajectory. If you are unhappy with your health or anything else in your life, you must address what's going on in your identity in order to change it long term.

To better understand how your identity may be influencing your current life experience, notice the words you choose when discussing health, relationships, and the world around you.

Even a simple little word like "my" can keep you stuck on the poor health trajectory.

For example:

- My anxiety
- My autoimmune disease
- My pain
- My Hashimoto's
- My brain fog

If you are using the word "my," it means you are taking ownership of that thing. And when we own something, the subconscious accepts it as part of who we are.

The things we claim ownership of are tied to us at a deeper level. If we lose one of these things, it can cause an identity conflict and trigger emotions such as grief, loss, regret, anger, fear.

This is why breakups, death, or changes in our relationship with something can feel like such a struggle. It may be why you might not be able to shake specific symptoms no matter how hard you've tried.

This also explains why you may have been able to follow a particular plan or process in the past and alleviate some of your symptoms, but then find you are back in the same place again just a few short weeks or months later. If your identity was anchored to that symptom or disease, or to a habit causing the symptom, unless you dissolve that identity anchor, the symptom will keep coming back like a boomerang.

Identity anchors are connections your subconscious has made to things that are familiar and "safe," even if they're actually hurting you. This means you will make decisions, without even realizing it, that are more likely to perpetuate that symptom or that health outcome because it's part of who you are.

One of our clients, Janet, said this during her very first health discovery call:

"I am an anxious person. I not a very good meditator. I can't sit still long enough to connect. I've always been this way. My mother used to tell everyone how much of a 'spirited child' I was. I started taking medication to control my anxiety when I was a teenager."

Based on this short description, what's Janet's identity? What are her core beliefs? What identity anchors do you notice that may be keeping her stuck?

Here are a few we noticed right away: She doesn't believe she is in control of her own body or that she is capable of even connecting with herself. The emotion or energy she feels has been labeled as "bad" (anxiety) which means it must be suppressed by something outside of herself (medication.) This belief was originated by her primary caregiver (mother), and was supported and reinforced by others, (at least her childhood doctor and current physician) since she was young.

Let's take a different perspective on Janet's story by shifting one belief controlling her identity:

What if Janet's feeling weren't anxiety and it was excitement instead? How could that influence her identity?

What if Janet believed she was capable of connecting with herself? How would that have changed her story?

What if Janet's mother had believed that "being spirited" was a good thing? How could that have impacted her life?

What if Janet's doctors had not prescribed medication to suppress her natural emotional response and taught her how to channel her energy differently? What change could that have had on her outcome?

After working with Janet to understand that her story was riddled with identity anchors and false truths, she realized that she ultimately had the power to change her belief of who she "really was," which dramatically impacted her symptoms, her gene expression, and health trajectory.

She is now off all of her anxiety and thyroid medications, her digestive problems are gone, she meditates easily and deeply, her sleep issues have subsided, and she no longer struggles with foggy brain or fatigue. Her relationship with her husband, which used to be strained, is enjoyable, and she feels connected with her two teen daughters.

Janet feels in control of her life now and doesn't look outside of herself to "fix" fractures in her soul. She knows how to communicate with her emotions and no longer sees symptoms as "bad." She simply sees them as messages and information helping her find her way to transformational healing.

What are you owning right now as part of "who you are?"

- Are you owing your illness?
- Are you owning your symptoms?
- Are you owning a situation in your life?
- What identity anchors are connected to your current health trajectory?
- Are you owning someone else's belief in what you are capable of?

Interestingly, the physical response in the body is remarkably the same for anxiety as it is for excitement. Increased heart rate, shortness of breath, butterflies in the stomach, racing thoughts, and inability to sleep. What determines the difference is whether you emotionally connect "good" or "bad" to the response. To change one to the other, you can simply change the word you choose to describe how you are feeling. Rather than saying, "I'm so anxious about this event," you can alter it to "I'm so excited about this event." Little conscious shifts like this will change your paradigm over time and help rewire connections to what is safe and what is dangerous.

Another way to uncover an identity connection controlling your life is to look at the ways you choose to describe yourself:

- I'm really good at compartmentalizing.
- I'm not an emotional person.
- I'm a perfectionist.
- I don't like change.
- I'm not really a crier.
- I've always been someone who doesn't socialize well.
- I hate traveling because I'm not good with new environments.
- I'm the kind of person who always attracts losers.
- Without me, everything falls apart.
- I'm the only one who can do things right.
- I'm the kind of person who suffers, so others don't have to.

Exercise

- Quickly write down the first three things that come to mind to finish this sentence:

    I'm the kind of person who...

- Quickly write the first three things that come to mind to finish this sentence:

    I'm not the kind of person who...

- Quickly write the first three things that come to mind

    It's my job to….

Exercise

Complete the missing parts of this sentence:

My _____ stops me from doing/having _____.

For example:

- My anxiety stops me from living fully.
- My foggy brain stops me from wanting to learn new things.
- My husband's lack of support stops me from having joy.

Now ask yourself: Are you ready to take ownership for what serves you and LET GO of ownership of what is not serving you?

Personal Identity Story - Kirstin

I grew up right outside of Philadelphia. I was raised by parents who did their best to raise me based on their interpretation of their life experiences, mixed with how their parents raised them filtered through their perspective of life experiences up to that point.

As discussed in the Science Section on epigenetics, my parents and the many generations before them passed along their beliefs, fears, traumas, and paradigms through genes as well as through behavioral conditioning.

When I was four years old, I was playing ball with my dad in the yard. Based on my father's conditioning from his family, boys were believed to be "better." In an effort to prepare me for a "man's world" my dad taught my sister and me early on how to adopt more stereotypical "boy-like" qualities, like honing athletic skills, not showing emotion, and being "strong."

On the front lawn of our house, balancing my dad's enormous baseball glove on my tiny hand, I prepared to catch the ball my father was about to throw to me. The ball left his hand, bounced off the leather glove, hit me in the face, and split my lip open.

As blood gushed down my chin and onto my favorite light blue unicorn and rainbow shirt, my father scooped me up and rushed me into the kitchen where my mom was making dinner. She saw me bleeding from the face, and quickly forgot about the roast she was preparing and exclaimed, "What happened?"

My dad was beaming. He was smiling ear to ear. He said, "Look at her. She's not crying!"

He was so proud.

My four-year-old developing subconscious mind which was eagerly searching for meaning and understanding in every moment, instantly absorbed the emotion and details of that incident and interpreted it all to mean, "Daddy loves me because I'm not crying." (I can still smell the mix of leather and oil from that perfectly worn-in glove whenever I recall that moment.)

My subconscious brain, now anchored to the smell of leather and the message that not crying was a good thing, (because it made my father proud, and proud fathers are more likely to pay attention to you, and when you are paid attention to, then you are more likely to be protected and safe) began watching closely every moment after that, looking for evidence that message was true.

At four years old, I locked down the idea that "Daddy pays attention to me when I'm not crying, when I don't show emotion, and when I am 'strong.'" My subconscious took that information and made it part of my paradigm which influenced my decisions, beliefs, and actions from that moment on.

I learned quickly how to behave like a strong, unemotional person. I used to pride myself on what a great "compartmentalizer" I was and how well I could handle nearly any situation without showing emotion. If you ever had a trauma, tragedy, or a tough day when you didn't cry or "get emotional," and you told that story to my dad, he would be so proud of you.

It makes sense now, looking back, how that belief, that one tiny moment in time, was so influential on major decisions in my life. Coupled with several other seemingly insignificant moments that formed my identity and belief of who I was and how I was "supposed to" show up in the world, these anchors impacted who I was friends with, what activities I participated in, how I handled pain (emotionally and physically), what limits I would push my body to, which college I chose, which guys I dated, and which ones I got serious with.

It explains why divorce was so traumatic for me, why I was so focused on my father's approval, and why I rebelled against my family by moving 1,500 miles away.

It also explains why I had so many stomach problems, migraines, and hormone imbalance. My body was speaking to me directly and I was ignoring it. I chose to white-knuckle through like the strong, emotionally controlled, powerful woman I thought I was supposed to be, all while my body attacked me from the inside.

This persisted until I finally chose to dig past the nutrition and the science roots of my symptoms and disease, and address the soul roots, too.

From the time we are born, our entire system is looking for messages to identify what will keep us safe. Be clear, however, that safe is not necessarily healthy or happy. We are wired to sense danger and stay alive.

In the first few years of life, our caregivers are the ones influencing these messages, which are also based on their experiences and beliefs of what has kept them safe.

Since your caregivers are the ones responsible to keep you alive and protect you from harm, you paid close attention to what made them pay attention to you, how they interacted with you, and what made them do things that made you feel safe. As discussed on Chapter 14: The Immune System, hardwired from birth is the fact there is a greater amount of safety in groups. So, learning how to be kept protected by "the tribe" is an important part of survival. If you go against the tribe, you could lose their protection, and the chances of surviving alone are low. So, we are hardwired to do, think, and behave as the tribe teaches us in order to stay alive through their protection. This is why it can be difficult to go against the beliefs of a group, especially when you are biologically connected to them.

So, if you've ever met someone and feel like you know them well, but then see them interact with their family and wonder, "Who the heck is this person?" you are seeing hardwiring, conditioning, and survival instincts kick in.

Chapter Takeaways

- Your identity drives your choices, decisions, and health trajectory. The words you choose are indicators of what you "identify" with and what may be keeping you stuck on a poor health trajectory.

- When your identity is anchored to a symptom or disease as "part of you," it may be anchoring that symptom or disease to you. Therefore, eliminating that issue may be creating underlying fear you are unsafe without it.

- Investigating how you describe yourself, what you think you are responsible for, and how you connect with your symptoms will give you incredible insight into why you haven't yet found your way onto your ideal health trajectory.

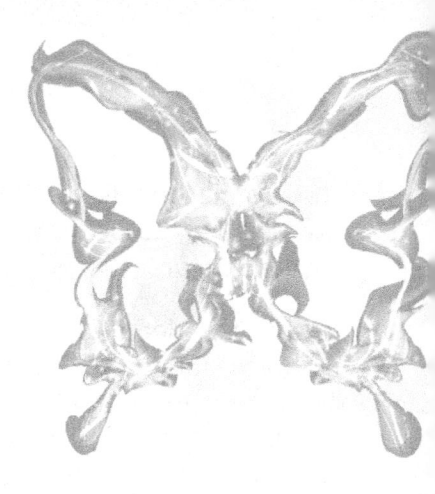

CHAPTER 22

PARADIGM & BELIEF

Thoughts, feelings, and beliefs formed before we were eight years old are what make up our paradigm. It's influenced by our families and main caregivers, our perceptions of the moments we experience, the vibration of energy around us, and our overall sense of safety and wellbeing. Your paradigm is a subconscious filter by which you judge every moment you experience and how you see yourself, and it is a powerful influence on everything that happens in your life. Every decision, action, and emotional reaction is impacted by your paradigm.

Belief, which is at the core of or your paradigm, is connected to every symptom, diagnosis, or problem you experience. Going back to the opening story about Meghan and her overactive thyroid, she made the choice to push off surgery because she believed she could heal, even when her doctor was telling her surgery was her only option. Her belief that healing was possible coupled with her willingness to change created the healing she experienced.

And that opportunity to heal is available to you, too.

To understand how the belief in your paradigm may be influencing your life, let's delve into The Pygmalion Effect and why it's so important to your healing trajectory.

The Pygmalion Effect is: **"When we expect certain behaviors of others, we are likely to act in ways that make the expected behavior more likely to occur."**

In a study titled "Teachers Expectations Can Influence How Students Perform" found at NPR.com, teachers were told that special testing could be determine which kids were likely to excel. The kids were then randomly selected and followed for two years. The kids who had been labeled most likely to excel ended up having the better test scores though the only difference being that the teachers believed those kids to be most likely to excel.

A similar study was done with doctors and their patients to see the impact the doctor's interaction with the patient had on the patient's reaction to treatment. The study can be found at Nature.com by searching "Socially Transmitted Placebo Effects" in their articles section.

In this study, when doctors believed they were giving patients a cream that would help their symptoms, the symptoms were more likely to go away then when the doctor thought they were giving the patient the actual medication, even when the cream was the placebo. When the doctor thought it was the placebo, there was less positive impact on the patient's symptoms even when it was the medical cream.

This study shows that the belief from the doctor was just as important, if not more so, to the patient's recovery. Therefore, it is critical to work with a practitioner who not only believes it's possible to heal, they also believe you have the possibility of healing, and that their recommended treatment is capable of being the tool that helps you get a positive outcome.

The impact a placebo can have on migraine pain can be found in the article called "Half A Drugs Power Comes from Thinking it Will Work" on NPR.com.

Whatever you believe to be true, influences your choices, actions, and ultimately, outcomes. The strength of belief, coupled with epigenetics is powerful. This means that you have incredible influence not only on yourself and your gene expression but also the gene expression of the people around you.

Also be clear that if you are working with a practitioner who doesn't believe you can heal, that can influence your outcome as well. Belief is powerful. Make sure that the people on your healing team not only believe you can heal, but they have worked with others who have also healed. This will raise the vibration of energy and belief, and increase your chances of activating transformational healing.

Chapter Takeaways

- Belief is a core component to healing. If you don't believe and/or the practitioner you are working with doesn't believe you can heal, then you're going to struggle to get on the ideal health trajectory.

- Teachers, parents, practitioners, and other leaders have incredible influence over outcomes. Use this information to help you achieve your goals and understand how important it is to surround yourself with people who believe in your success.

- Dozens of studies have been done on The Pygmalion Effect and Placebo Effect supporting how powerful belief is on outcome. When you believe something (positive or negative), it is much more likely that result will occur.

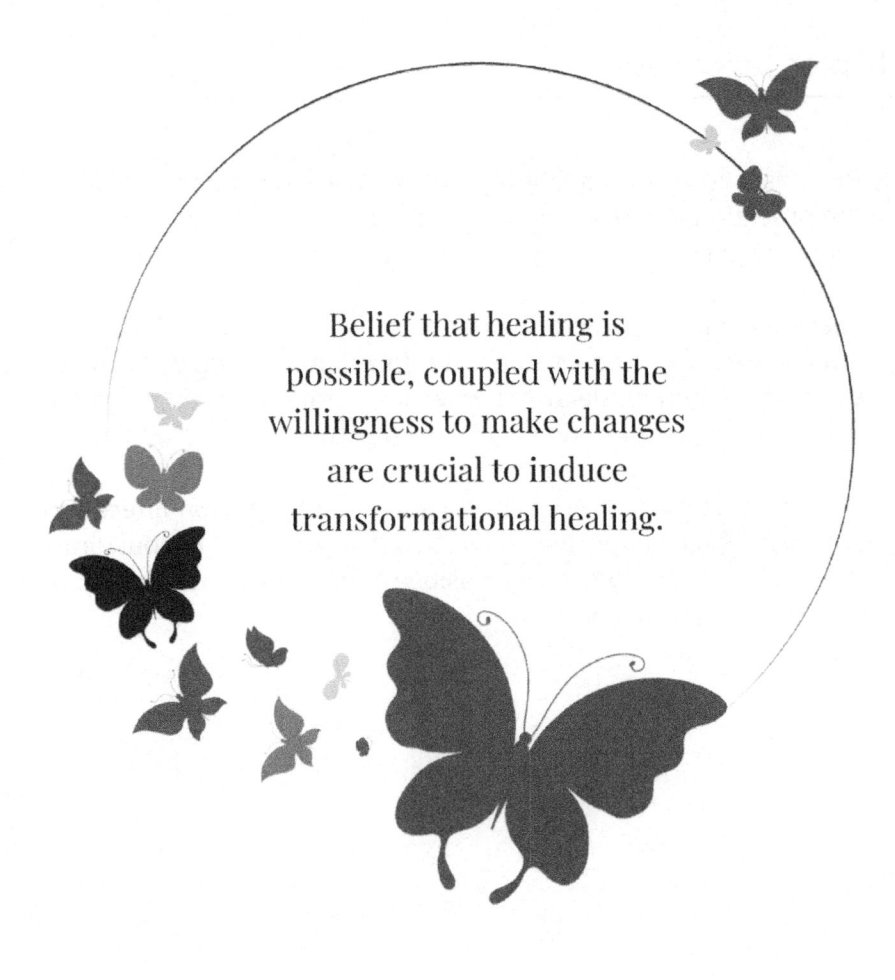

Belief that healing is possible, coupled with the willingness to make changes are crucial to induce transformational healing.

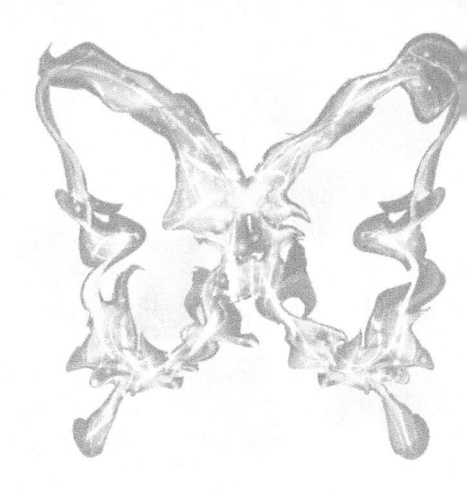

CHAPTER 23

NEGATIVE VS POSITIVE TRAUMA

The story of Kirstin when she was four years old, splitting her lip open playing ball with her father is an example of a "positive trauma." A positive trauma is a shocking moment that locks into the paradigm and triggers a perceived positive experience, but causes a long-term negative result. Getting hit in the face with the ball was a shocking experience and could have easily become a negative trauma, but because of Kirstin's dad's positive reaction to her perceived lack of emotion, her subconscious recorded it as a positive experience.

Since the experience created a positive connection for Kirstin, she looked for ways to reinforce it because she connected it to a feeling of safety and protection from her tribe. But over time, this also stopped her from connecting effectively with her emotions and process them in a healthy way.

Experiences are interpreted as either positive or negative based on our perception, which is influenced by our paradigm. Our paradigm is created through epigenetics; nurturing and conditioning from our family, friends, and environment; our hardwired connections to what we think is "safe"; and our perception of our experiences.

A large majority (if not all) of our paradigm is anchored into our subconscious by the time we are about seven years old.

Significant experiences anchor into our system and shape (or reinforce) our paradigm the same way. When an emotional response is triggered, it is recorded first by our cells and tissues and then is recorded by the brain. Instantly, based on past experiences, conditioning, or reactions from the people around us, that emotional response is determined to be a "positive" experience or a "negative" one. The physical and mental responses are then also recorded into memory and anchored to the emotional response.

That memory is then locked into our body emotionally, mentally, and physically and can be recalled quickly when triggered by a similar event. Though it's only typically labeled as "a trauma" when a person's emotional response appears on the surface to be "a distressing experience," both positive and negative anchors influence the body subconsciously the same way. We challenge the traditional definition of a trauma because it doesn't account for significant experiences the body interprets as positive but cause a long-term negative impact.

A heightened emotional moment interpreted positively or negatively still enters the system the same way: through the cells and tissues first, and then gets recorded in the memory. It's then put through the paradigm's filter to determine if the experience is negative or positive. If it's interpreted as negative, the experience is then anchored to feelings of fear and anxiety, which release chemicals triggering a flight or fight response. If it's interpreted as positive, the experience is then anchored to feelings of safety, which release chemicals of joy and elation. But that doesn't mean the positive experience was healthy or that the connection isn't harmful long term.

In fact, the "positive traumas" can often cause deeper-rooted issues, as people find themselves "chasing" that positive feeling of safety or elation.

This is when you see people chasing things such as:

- Perfectionism.
- Control.
- Over-support of others (aka "Florence Nightingale syndrome").
- Performance syndrome (chasing the "win" or accolade and feeling

let down once they reach that goal).

- Ignoring symptoms such as pain, exhaustion, or brain fog in an attempt to feel powerful, "hard working," or "able to push through."

From our experience, the root cause of these issues is connected to a "positive trauma" early in life that was connected to a moment or series of moments that reinforced safety, but may now cause feelings of scarcity, fear, abandonment, resentment, or loss of control.

This is exactly what ended up happening to Kirstin. Not surprisingly, her attempts to reinforce the positive anchor made to suppressing emotions and making her father proud, ended up causing digestive issues and an inner conflict with her true Self, who is a deeply emotional person.

Chapter Takeaways

- Your belief is connected to every one of your symptoms, diagnosis, or problems.

- Positive trauma can be even more detrimental to health than negative trauma because typically, we purposely reinforce positive trauma.

- Understanding the moments in your life which had a profound impact will help you better understand why you perceive life the way you do. This understanding gives insight into how to shift onto your ideal health trajectory and change your current life experience.

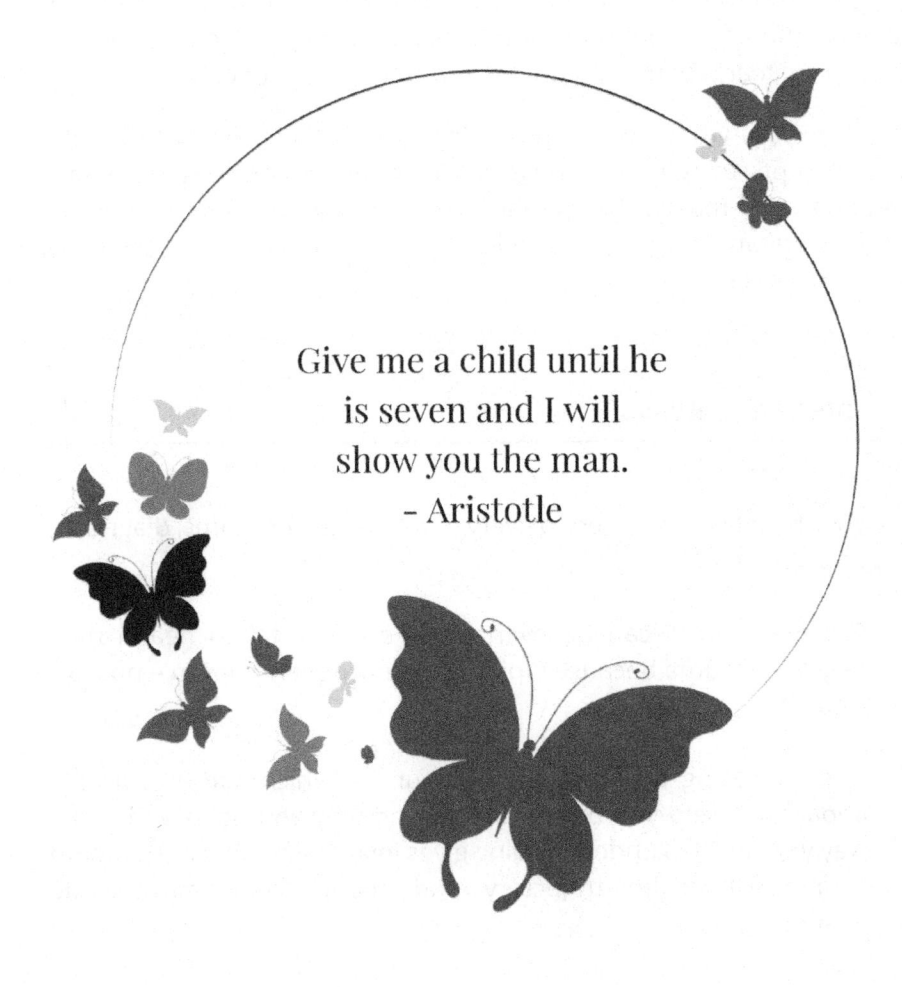

> Give me a child until he
> is seven and I will
> show you the man.
> - Aristotle

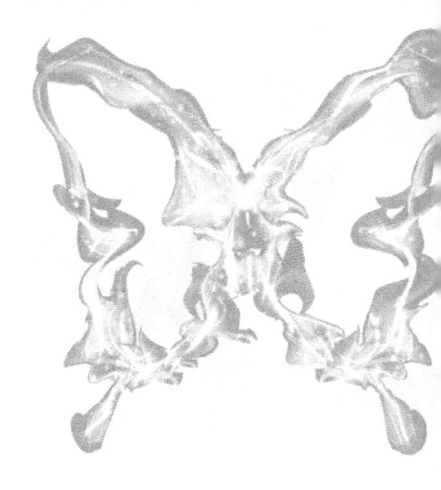

CHAPTER 24

WOUNDED CHILDREN

Hidden traumas may be controlling your ability to heal. Something that could have happened to you at four years old may still be having an impact 20, 30, or 50 years later. Just as Kirstin's decisions and beliefs were driven by her four-year-old self in her story about playing catch with her dad, her need to "make daddy proud" by suppressing emotions was still driving her decisions for decades.

Those trauma moments (positive or negative) create underlying "wounded children" which influence how your adult self makes decisions based on the fears of the wounded child, which don't necessarily line up with your ideal health trajectory. If you're on a trajectory of poor health, even though you feel like you've been doing "all the right things" but cannot seem to get better, it's guaranteed there is a wounded child (or two or five) in control.

If you've ever interacted with little kids, you know they are not making decisions logically and weighing out all the options. Kids make decisions based on their emotional vibration. That's it.

This is why you may find yourself acting like a child when you're in a triggered moment. It's as if you are instantly transported back to being that child where the "wound" originated and that shocking moment occurred.

If the wound isn't addressed and that wounded child doesn't feel safe, she will continue to take over whenever she senses danger.

Exercise

Let's get some insight into where you may have some wounded children lurking about.

Take a moment right now and think about a time where you felt triggered, deeply upset, or quickly angered. Perhaps it was the last argument you had with a spouse or family member, especially if the core of the argument seems to occur frequently with no resolve. Typically, those types of arguments are really about something deeper than what started the argument, and there's usually a "wounded child" who has stepped in and is fighting because she feels unsafe.

HACK:

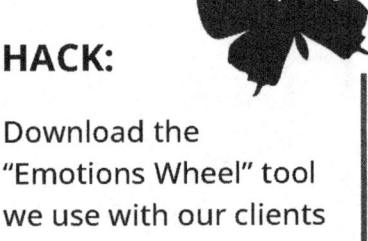

Download the "Emotions Wheel" tool we use with our clients to help them access hidden emotions and get a better understanding of their wounded children at www.nourish123.com/thbonus

Now, take a deep breath and see if you can "step back" from that argument and look at it as objectively and calmly as you can. What was the argument really about? What was the clearest emotion you were feeling during the triggered experience? Was it embarrassment, shame, fear, confusion, abandonment, guilt, jealously, betrayal, stupidity, insecurity, overwhelm, helplessness, hopelessness, oppression?

Choose a word, or a few words that explain how you felt in that moment. Now, when was the first time (or the most significant time) you remember feeling that way?

What else was going on in that moment?

Can you think of another moment, maybe the earliest one when you also felt that way?

What did the you in that moment really want? Why was she feeling the ways she was? Why did she behave like that?

Was she feeling unheard, unnoticed, or unimportant? Which need, or needs weren't being met?

We have a process to help flesh out wounded children. It also helps clients then interpret what the child felt she was missing, and heal the wound from that experience.

You can use a similar process now, by spending some time understanding that wounded child, what she needed, and why she continues to appear in your life.

We've found that it's incredibly helpful to name the wounded child and truly see her, acknowledged her, and give her what she needs so she doesn't continue to show up in such a dramatic way. Imagine what she looks like and what she would be wearing. How old is she? What's her favorite thing? What does she want the most? What does she believe about herself and the world around her? Really spend some time getting to know her so she feels valid and seen. That's all most people really want, right?

When you better understand the wounded child, it will shed lots of insight on your reactions to certain situations and people, why you may be experiencing specific symptoms, and what you can do to start creating more balance in your life.

And as we've discussed before, every single decision is made by the paradigm formed when we are young. This means that your wounded children are connected to your paradigm.

If you cannot imagine reaching the goal you say you want, or the wounded child thinks it's dangerous to pursue, then the goal will be out of reach. If you do not believe healing is possible, then you can repeat positive affirmations and mantras all day long and they won't solve your health issues.

Repeating over and over, "I am thin! I am thin! I am thin!" won't make a bit of difference if you cannot envision yourself at a healthy weight, or if your wounded child feels safer holding onto excess weight.

This is where positive thinking and mantras go horribly wrong and often *reinforce* the underlying core fears causing the symptoms. If you don't address the underlying belief of "I am not good enough" or "I'm not lovable" stemming from your wounded child, and you keep repeating a mantra that triggers those negative beliefs, then you will trigger the wounded child and reinforce the negative belief every time you say the positive one.

Addressing the needs of the wounded child can change your entire trajectory and get you on the path to healing.

Remember the story about Lori whose body was holding onto extra weight to protect her from "starving?" Under that fear, was a wounded child who felt abandoned, unimportant, and dismissed by her parents. It's that wounded child who was further traumatized by her husband leaving and why that experience pushed her into feeling more fear.

Until the underlying fear was surfaced, and the wounded child anchored to that fear was comforted, Lori's subconscious kept her protected by holding onto the added pounds. When you are aware of why your body behaves the way it does, and what the symptoms are trying to tell you, then you can be in charge and process the hidden issues.

Chapter Takeaways

- Wounded child perceptions influence your identity and paradigms, which override your balanced adult self and the decisions you make.

- When we are triggered by anxiety, rage, and panic, it is typically an underlying wounded child screaming that they don't feel safe and need to be seen, witnessed, and heard.

- Positive thinking and positive mantras can actually reinforce underlying core fears if the wounded child's needs are left unaddressed.

Who is your most predominant wounded child?

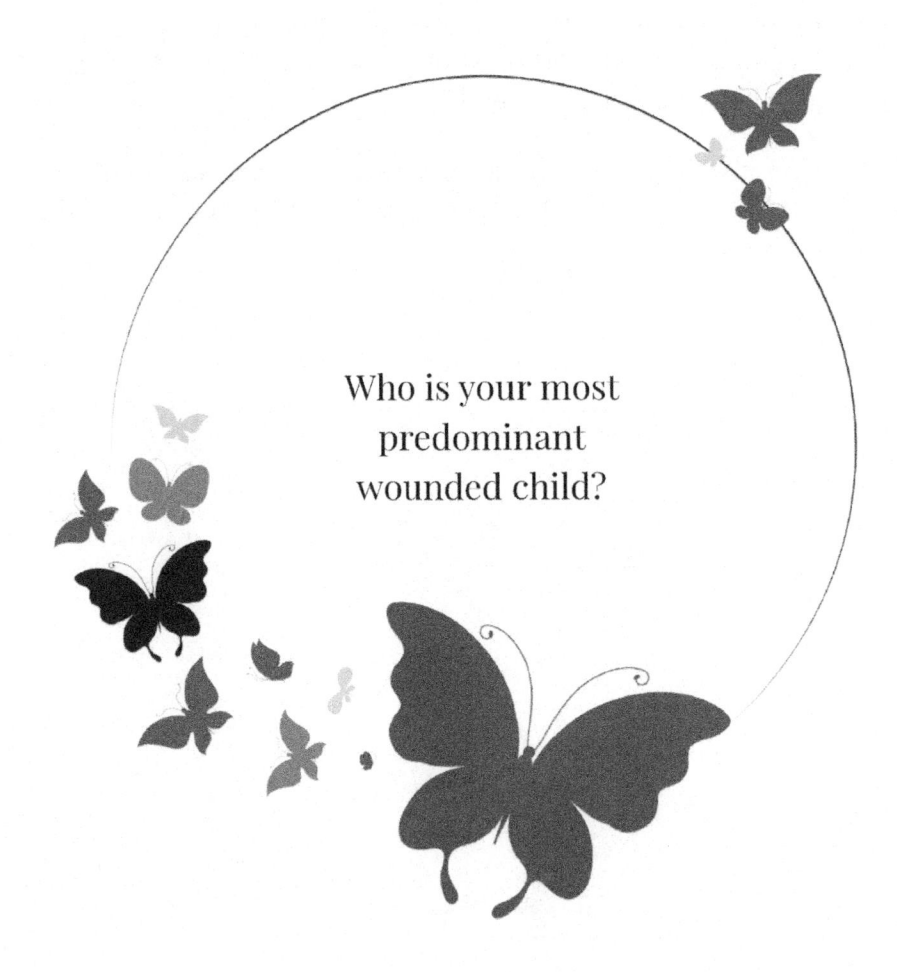

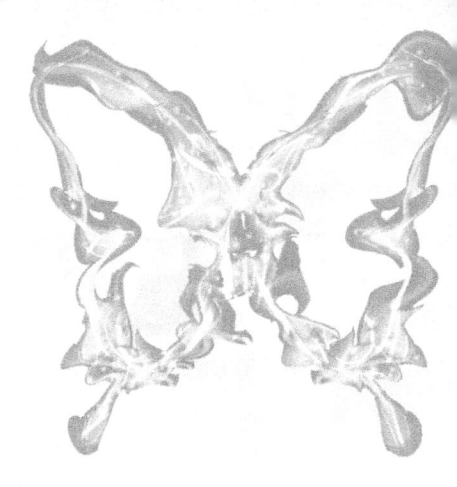

CHAPTER 25

SYMPTOMS ARE A MESSAGE

All of your symptoms and the way they present mean something to your body.

When you feel pain, stress, insomnia, or gas, do you think about the emotional and physical connection between your body and the symptom you are experiencing? Do you run to the medicine cabinet and try to suppress that symptom without addressing it? Do you simply ignore the symptom and hope it goes away?

Understanding your symptoms is the bridge to your ideal health trajectory and transformational healing.

When symptoms are ignored or suppressed, the body will look for alternative ways to communicate with you. Over time, these messages will get more dramatic and forceful in an attempt to get your attention and alert you to underlying imbalances such as resentment, shame, fear, and discontent.

The body is constantly communicating. Every symptom, every ache, and every reaction is the body's way of telling us something is out of balance and needs attention. It's up to you to interpret that communication and give your body what it's asking for to find balance.

Let's shed some light on the possible messages your body is trying to send you by helping to translate a few of the most common symptom connections.

Headaches

Headaches are often the body's way of saying "You are disconnected. You are not paying attention to me." This symptom is a way for your system to let you know your ability to connect with yourself deeply is fractured or completely nonexistent. If you are a master compartmentalizer, then you are probably struggling to connect your symptoms to their underlying soul root cause. You may, in fact, struggle with this section altogether and argue that you are totally in control of your emotional life. This means you are trying to "logic your way through" your solution. And you've probably spent lots of time, effort, money, and energy focused on the Nutrition (food, diet, supplements, fitness) and the Science (labs, diagnosis, physiology, genetics) part of the journey and pushed the Soul piece to the side.

Digestive Distress

Stomach pain and distress are often red flags alerting you to internal conflict about who you are, who you were "supposed to be," and what is happening in your life. Your inability to "digest life" is often directly connected to how you feel about yourself, your identity, and how you fit into the world around you. This identity conflict can often be the root cause of autoimmune (self-attack) related issues. Stomach problems are an indicator that your paradigm is being challenged.

Thyroid Issues

According to the American Thyroid Association, 20 million Americans have some form of thyroid disease. Levothyroxine was the second most commonly prescribed medication in the entire United States in 2019, and one out of eight women will experience thyroid disorder in their lifetime.

A common underlying root cause for people with thyroid problems is related to how they communicate with others (and themselves) about their needs, desires, and purpose.

They hold back from "speaking their truth." By not expressing this truth, it gets caught in the throat and festers, demanding to be let go. The more you hold back and deny your truth and the person you truly are in your soul, the more ways your body will fight back and demand freedom of expression.

If you feel that you are not freely expressing yourself, that you are not living your true purpose, or you are suppressing your ability to communicate to yourself and to the world who you really are, then this may be an underlying root cause of your thyroid-related dysfunction.

This issue also extends to symptoms associated with the throat, sinuses, neck, jaw, gums, teeth, shoulders, neck, thyroid, and the parathyroid, which are all located near the thyroid.

Physically, people will often walk with their head down or shoulders hunched forward in an effort to close off and protecting their throat area. They hold back and don't express themselves openly or they overexpress and have no filter and talk excessively. They often hold their hands over their throats, touch their neck when they speak, or even hold their hands close to or over their mouths.

When the thyroid is out of balance, it often shows up as:

- "Being too open" - Overtalking, dogmatic, self-righteous, arrogance, inability to listen to others or consider alternate opinions. This is often a good sign that the thyroid is "hyper" or too much thyroid medication is being taken.

- "Being too blocked" - Holds back from self-expression, unreliable, holds inconsistent views, overly quiet, coughs or clears throat before speaking. This is also a sign that the thyroid is "hypo," and the thyroid isn't communicating effectively with the pituitary gland.

People who are connected express themselves in a balanced way and are typically good communicators, contented, connect easily through meditation or prayer, often artistically inspired, and are able to communicate who they are and what they need effectively. They are also good listeners and connectors with others in addition to themselves.

Autoimmune Disease

Internal conflict causes imbalance and fear in the system as the soul fights to be seen and heard. When you are in conflict with your core identity or trying to be who you think you are "supposed to be" rather than who you really are, that creates an internal war.

Hashimoto's or Graves' disease, means your immune system is attacking your thyroid, causing it to have a hypothyroid or hyperthyroid response.

Celiac disease is the immune system attacking the lining of the gut. Vitiligo is the immune system attacking the pigment of the skin.

So, the question is: Why would your immune system (which is designed to protect you and help you heal) attack part of you?

When your immune system doesn't recognize something within the body, it often responds by attacking what it can't identify as part of Self, out of fear that it is dangerous.

When you don't speak your truth and stifle your feelings and beliefs, this means you aren't expressing your true YOU. Over time, the body becomes confused and in conflict with you and how you express Self.

This conflict creates fear and confusion between what is part of Self and what is the enemy. Your immune system, in an attempt to protect you from harm, will attack anything seen as dangerous or not part of Self. By not fully expressing what makes you YOU or not accepting your true Self, you are triggering the immune system to start its attack in an attempt to protect you from what it doesn't recognize.

Are you now making a stronger connection between autoimmune disease (the body attacking itself) and the suppression of expression of your true desire and purpose?

Heart

The heart is so much more than an organ that pumps blood. It's a central connector to the body physically, energetically, emotionally, and spiritually. And it often gives incredible information on healing when you know what to look for.

A few years ago, heart issues were reclassified as an autoimmune condition, and heart disease is a leading cause of death for men and women all around the world, but especially in the United States.

Whenever we work with a client who has any heart or circulatory related issue, we immediately look for other indicators of "heart pain." Issues such as abandonment, shame, loneliness, grief, and lack of self-love. Learning to love Self, feel a sense of belonging to a tribe, and release underlying emotional wounds can dramatically impact healing.

Here are some amazing details about the heart, that may shed some light on why the heart is more than just a physical organ, and how it has so much impact on transformational healing.

- Of all your organs, the heart never gets to rest making it the organ with the most mitochondria per cell in the body.
- The heart beat is self-initiated from within the heart with no reliance on the brain.
- The heart can be removed and placed in a salt solution, where it will continue to beat on its own.
- The heart begins beating at three weeks after conception, even though the brain isn't formed until about week six.
- Heart cells stop dividing, which means heart cancer is extremely rare.
- Laughing is good for your heart. It reduces stress and gives a boost to your immune system.
- The heart and brain have more nerve connections to each other than any other system in the body. This gives insight on the direct connection to why what you think has such an incredible impact on how your heart functions, what you feel emotionally, and why people associate love and pain with the heart.
- The heart's electromagnetic frequency is about 60 times stronger than that of the brain.
- According to Chinese medicine, the oldest medicine on Earth, the heart, small intestine, and thymus gland are all directly connected.
- The heart's strength can be heard in the voice. Voice characteristics such as pitch, amplitude, cracking, and sounding unsure can help uncover heart disruptions.
- When we are stressed, it effects the heart beat which will beat in a "disconnected" way and makes us feel out of balance, anxious, and disjointed.
- With about 75% accuracy, science can predict what someone is feeling by looking at their heart beat activity using heart rate variability analysis.

https://www.ncbi.nlm.nih.gov/pmc/articles/PMC4311559/

Did you know that "broken heart syndrome" (also known as takotsubo cardiomyopathy) is an actual medical diagnosis which has similar symptoms to a heart attack. Takotsubo cardiomyopathy is caused by a rush of stress hormones from an emotional or physical stress event. During the stress event, and often long after it, people feel unworthy of receiving joy, love, or happiness and become resistant to change and accept defeat more easily. These energy draining reactions impact gene expression and keep people stuck on a poor health trajectory.

Chapter Takeaways

- Every symptom and the exact way they express means something specific to your body. Understanding the story your symptoms are telling is the bridge to your healing path and transformational healing.

- If you ignore or suppress symptoms, your body will find alternative ways of communicating with you until it gets your attention.

- When you learn to decipher your body's way of communicating, it will open a whole new level of healing you cannot access any other way.

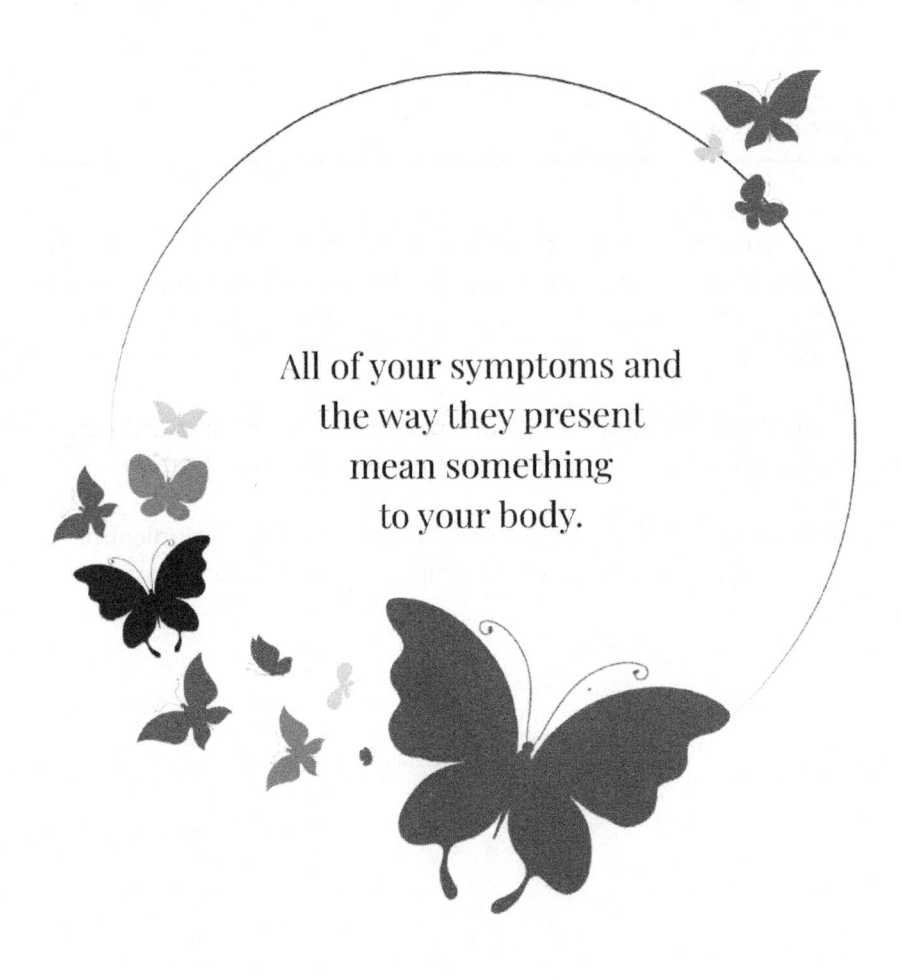

All of your symptoms and
the way they present
mean something
to your body.

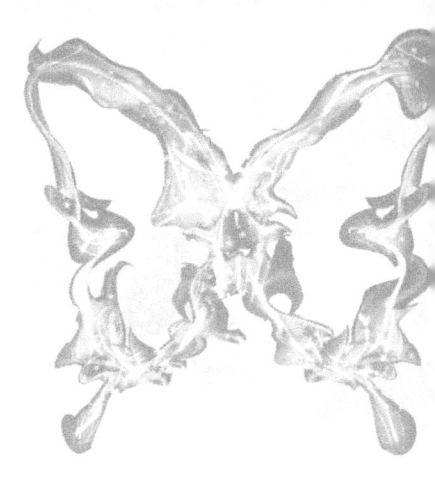

CHAPTER 26

INTERPRETING SYMPTOMS

Every symptom means something to you specifically. If you shift your perspective and see the symptom as *a gift* alerting you to help you feel better, connect more deeply, and achieve greater fulfillment, how would that change your current experience?

A great way to unravel this message and see the gift is to ask:

- Why are my symptoms mine?
- Why are they happening to me in this specific way, now?
- What could the message be that my body is trying to bring to my attention?
- What direct impact have the symptoms had on my life?
- What are they stopping me from doing?
- What indirect (or direct) signals are these symptoms sending me?
- What indirect (or direct) impact are the symptoms having on my life, goals, and relationships?

Do your best to answer these questions with as little judgment as possible. The goal isn't to find "all the things you're doing wrong," it's to shed light into the shadows of your paradigm and get access to information that will give you the awareness you need to change your current health trajectory.

Allow yourself to "feel the feels" and connect with the emotions that surface, even if your instinct is to disengage, toss the questions aside, or shove the feelings down. This is a sign that there is something deeper connected to your symptoms, and this is your chance to glean some important insight.

On the flip side, don't stay stuck in the pain of the emotion that surfaces. Use the emotional connection to help you make the shift you need to step forward and change your current trajectory. Ask yourself, "What will compel me to do things differently than I'm doing right now?"

The thought process, the patterns, and the decisions that got you where you are now must change to reach a new level of healing. Though you may feel energized when you decide to change your trajectory, you also may feel fear or doubt. Change can feel scary to the warm safe comfort of familiar patterns.

Those patterns can be so comfortable that your body may intentionally keep you stuck in your pain, fatigue, and anxiety. These symptoms may be so familiar, the subconscious thinks they are safe. Don't underestimate the power of what is familiar.

Chapter Takeaways

- Shift your perspective and see your symptoms as a gift showing you the healing path, rather than a curse to keep you from healing. This will enable a deeper connection with who you are, and how your body communicates what it needs to feel safe, balanced, and free.

- When you can be curious and ask yourself questions without judgement, it helps surface the messages beneath the symptoms.

- Allowing yourself to connect with the emotion tied to each symptom can also help you understand if there is a wounded child attached to the symptom and shed light on the emotional root cause of the symptom.

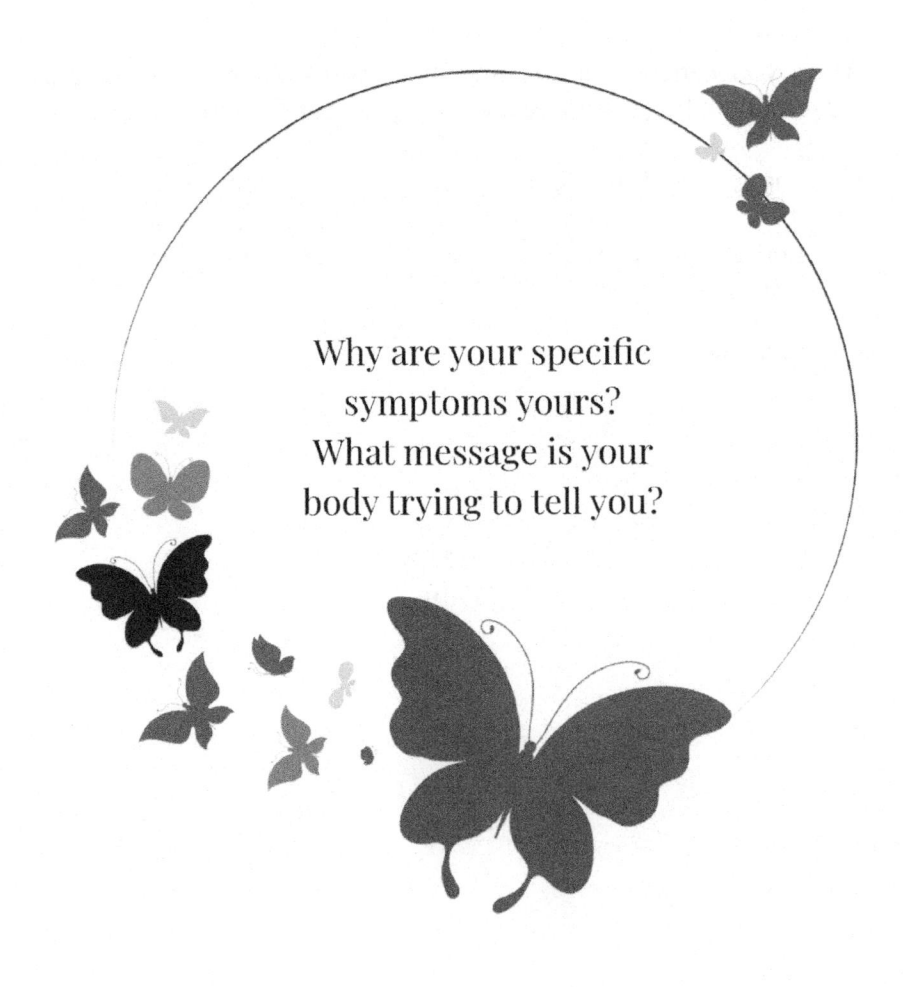

Why are your specific
symptoms yours?
What message is your
body trying to tell you?

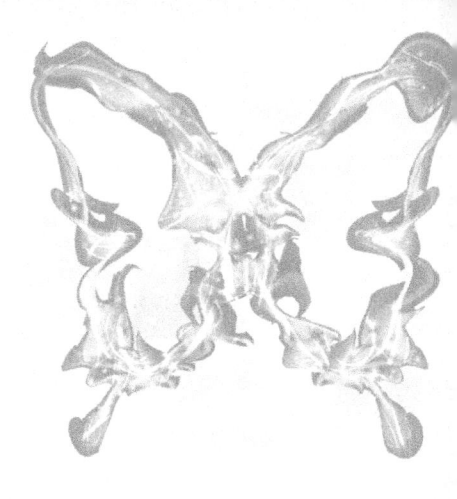

CHAPTER 27

YOUR FILTER & FAMILIAR PATTERNS

The paradigm in your subconscious uses your past as a filter for all of your current and future decisions. One of the most influential reasons for making any decision is based on how "safe" or familiar the decision feels.

Therefore, if you are used to life always feeling "so freaking hard", anytime it feels like things are going too smoothly, you question it. Then your paradigm pushes you to make a decision that, in turn, makes life feel hard again.

How often do the people around say things like:

- Life is hard and then you die.
- Marriage is a struggle, and you have to fight to stay together.
- If it isn't difficult, it's not worth doing.
- The struggle makes the reward sweeter.
- Anything worth having is worth fighting for.
- No pain, no gain.

If you grew up with one or more caregivers who were alcoholics, substance abusers, perfectionists, narcissists, control freaks, emotionally shut down, emotionally unstable, or physically, verbally, sexually, or emotionally abusive, or there was no stable energy in your life, then chaos may feel safe to you.

Look around your life. Is it chaotic? Does it always feel like you can't catch a break? Are you constantly rushing from one thing to the next and waiting for "the other shoe to drop?" Does it seem that nothing is ever calm and everyone around you is barely holding it together?

If chaos is familiar or expected, there is a frequency your paradigm is sending attracting that chaos to you because it feels safer to be in chaos than to be out of it.

> **HACK:**
>
> When using "absolute" language such as always, never, must, all, none, completely, and perfect there is typically a wounded child in charge. Balanced adults don't have unrealistic expectations or make demands the way a wounded child does. Watch for phrases that use absolute language like, "You always do this!" or "I never get a break around here!" so you can become more aware of potential wounded child moments.

Jeanie's Story

Jeanie has a pattern. Every time she begins to make progress, within a few weeks, she shows up for a coaching meeting and launches into 25 minutes of stories about how everyone around her is failing to meet her expectations, how challenging life is, and how "unexpected" things keep getting in the way of her success.

Her husband keeps bringing home junk foods, which she knows make her feel bad when she eats them, but she does it anyway. Her children never seem to be able to follow through on their responsibilities around the house, putting more work on her, and her best friend

Chapter 27 – Your Filter & Familiar Patterns | 167

always seems to have some sort of personal crisis, which causes her to drop everything and run to her friend's rescue.

The teachers at her kids' school are always assigning last minute projects, the people at church are lousy at following through on their promises to help with the fund-raising events Jeanie is the chairperson for, and her siblings don't help as much with taking care of her aging parents as she does.

According to Jeanie, despite her best efforts to stay on track with her nutrition, workout schedule, and soul homework, the people in her life keep making bad choices causing her to have to pick up the slack and get thrown off her healing trajectory.

Jeanie says she's frustrated and tired of yelling at everyone to simply do what they are expected to do. She feels that her health is declining because she cannot rely on anyone but herself and doesn't get the support she needs. Her symptoms suddenly start piling up again, and her limited time is being eaten away by running to urgent care for a broken toe, strep throat, and an aggressive case of shingles.

In one week, her washer broke, one of the family cars was damaged in a parking lot while they were in the mall, and her son's backpack was stolen at a football rally.

"It's always something!" Jeanie said. "No matter how hard I try, I can't get ahead."

Obviously, there are several layers to Jeanie's story, but what common threads do you see in this description of her interpretation of events. What does it tell you about her perceptions, beliefs, identity anchors, and expectations?

How are those perceptions, beliefs, anchors, and expectations creating Jeanie's pattern of finally getting on the right healing trajectory just to be pulled off it in a few weeks? What might Jeanie actually be afraid of, causing her to feel safer when everything is in chaos around her, and no one seems to be a reliable **source of support?**

It's typically much easier to see emotional patterns when analyzing someone else's story than your own because you aren't connected to the triggers and wounds which created the patterns and caused the paradigm. We work with clients to teach them techniques and processes to recognize, surface, and rewire these controlling paradigms and change their perceptions so they can alter their life experiences and get on their ideal healing trajectory.

Chapter Takeaways

- Your paradigm determines how you behave and what decisions you make based on how "safe" or familiar the decision feels.

- When you are familiar with struggle and challenge, you are more likely to choose the path that feels most difficult and question the one which feels "too easy" even if you say you really want to live a more simple and easy life.

- Scan your life and see what familiar patterns appear. Those familiar patterns are happening because it's part of your paradigm and belief system that those patterns have kept you safe.

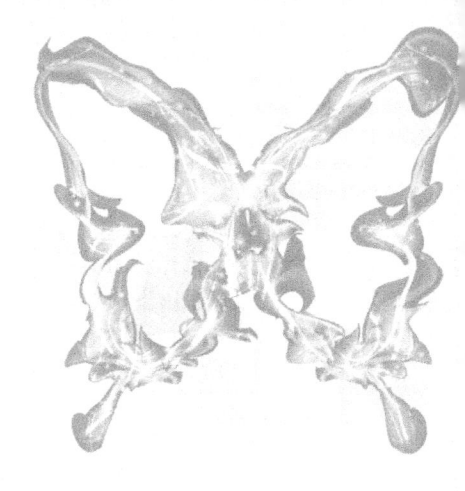

CHAPTER 28

YOUR PARADIGM ISN'T LOGICAL (AND NEITHER ARE YOU)

Logically, you can say it would be better if you weren't living in chaos, but your paradigm doesn't make decisions logically.

In fact, no decision you ever make is being made from logic. They are all driven by emotions.

Guarantee that last paragraph ruffled some feathers. As much as many of us would like to believe that we are making decisions with pure logic and no emotion, every single decision is being driven by an emotion. This isn't an opinion. This is how we are all wired.

Decisions are emotionally based on values, which are part of your paradigm along with past experiences, conditioning, and beliefs. We simply use logic *to justify* the decision.

So, if you don't understand your emotional drivers, then you will be confused as to why you are continuing to get the results you get. Fears will rule every decision you make in an attempt to keep you safe in the familiar.

By understanding your drivers, you will better understand what is influencing your decisions, beliefs, and actions and what impact that has on the trajectory of your health and your life experiences.

When these drivers are hidden, they control your life without you knowing, which takes away your ability to do anything about it. It's like walking into the house and knowing that something just doesn't smell right. You look in the trash, the laundry, the dishwasher, and in the bathroom. After days of searching and the smell getting more pronounced, you finally discover that a sweet potato rolled behind the refrigerator and was rotting back there.

Just because you now know the root cause of the smell, doesn't mean the smell instantly disappears. You actually have to do something about it, or it will get worse as it festers and attracts insects and vermin.

Even though it won't be pleasant, you have to deal with it, and clean up the mess.

Just as the smell was a sign alerting you there was a problem, all your symptoms (even any diagnosis you have) are also alerts telling you, "Hey, there's something going on here that needs your attention." That's it.

If you ignore those signs, alerts, or symptoms (the headache, fatigue, foggy brain, belly weight, anxiety) they don't just go away.

And even if you notice the alert, and you are prepared to do something about it, if you aren't looking in the right place for the root cause, you won't be able to find it.

What we can tell you with certainty is that root causes aren't typically corrected by a one-size-fits-all magic diet, $400 a month of supplements, or $9,000 of labs looking for the unicorn diagnosis. Though custom nutrition, supplementation, and labs can help aid your healing process, the deepest root cause solutions are typically hiding in the shadows of your paradigm.

Learning to rewire the underlying traumas stopping you from connecting to who you really are and expressing your true Self, is one of the most important pieces to healing, no matter what the issue or symptom, and most especially when dealing with thyroid, chronic illness, and autoimmune related challenges.

Chapter Takeaways

- Decisions are made emotionally based on values, beliefs, and experiences hidden in your paradigm. Logic is then used to justify the decision.

- Understanding what is driving your values and influencing your decisions will help you get on the health trajectory you want and not feel tied to the one you don't want.

- Though it often feels unpleasant and even frightening to surface underlying drivers, they need to be addressed to be free from them.

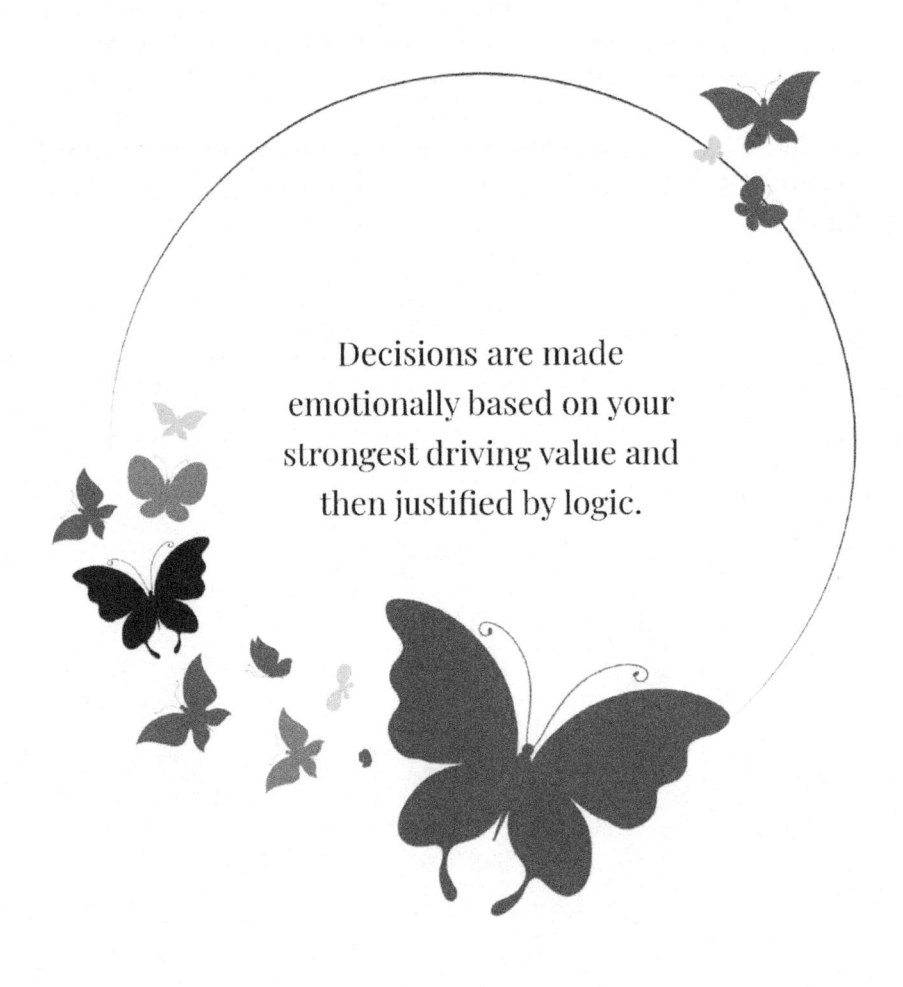

Decisions are made emotionally based on your strongest driving value and then justified by logic.

PART 5

THE PLAN

We all have blocks and hidden challenges deep in the subconscious. Learning how to identify those hurdles, surface them, and rewire them is critical to healing.

In the next several sections you will learn how to locate some of those hidden blocks, how to interpret what they mean, and some strategies and techniques to dissolve them.

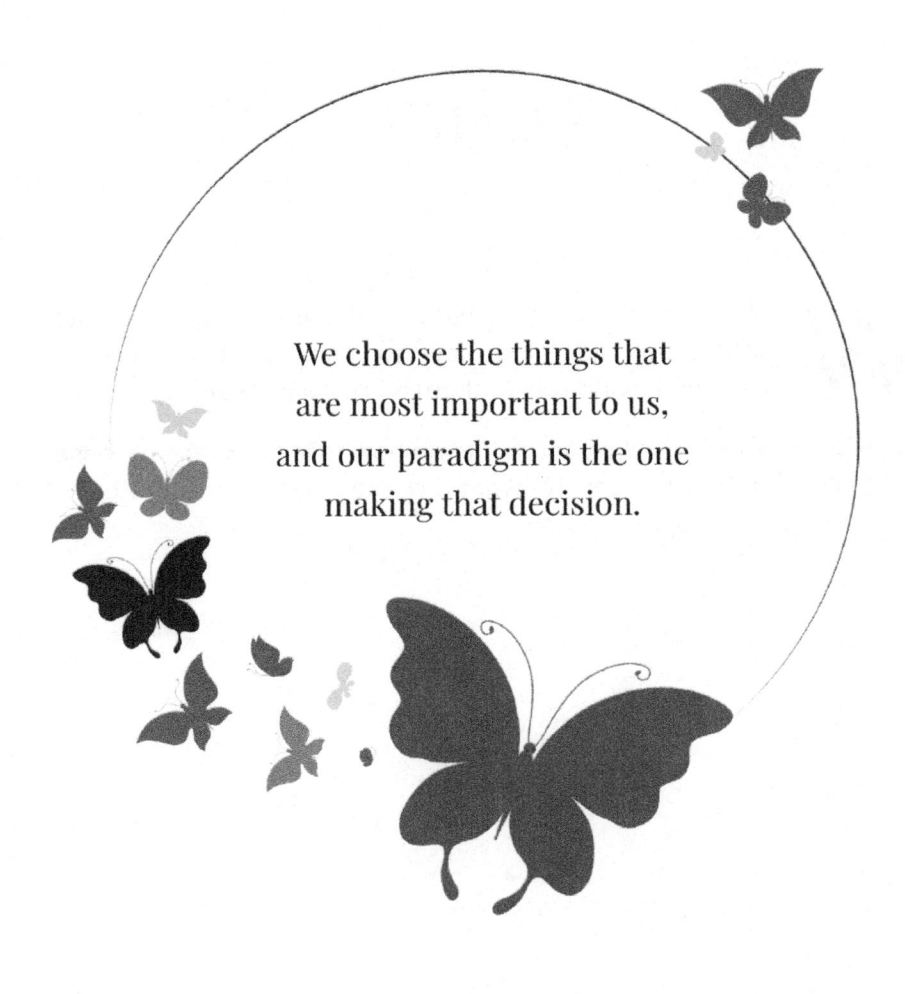

> We choose the things that are most important to us, and our paradigm is the one making that decision.

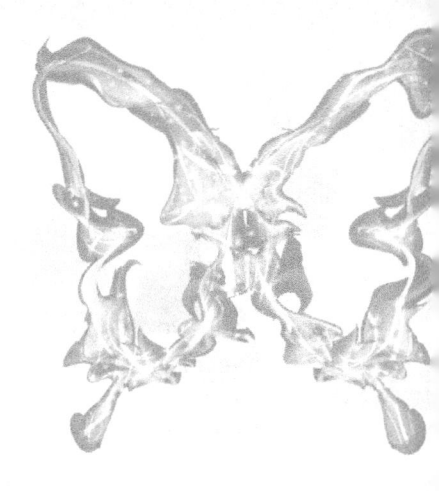

CHAPTER 29

IDENTIFYING HURDLES TO HEALING

Some of our clients feel better within just a few days and even a few hours after enrolling in our program. They haven't seen their nutrition strategy yet. They haven't gotten their lab results back yet. They haven't even logged into the client system yet. So, why would somebody feel instantaneously better the moment they became a client?

For some, it's because they finally made a decision, and took action to put themselves first, and their body realized that they were finally on the right path. For others, it's because it's the first time they felt heard, supported, and understood. And for some, it's because they let go of the fear and shifted to a new paradigm of belief that there was a better way to live. As we discussed in Chapter 22: Paradigm and Belief, belief is a powerful driver which can single handedly alter your health and your life experience.

If you're hesitating to step forward and claim your health, it's an opportunity for you to uncover a block keeping you stuck. Any excuse preventing you from stopping the cycle and getting the tools and support you need to move on to your ideal health trajectory, that's a glimmer into your subconscious that believes you are safer by sticking with the status quo than doing something different.

Knowing how the subconscious hardwiring works lets you see that any reason you have for not moving forward to claim your ideal health is a sign your desire to heal ranks lower on your priority list than you may realize. This is not an opinion. It's not a judgment. It's just the way our brains work.

When we have a choice, whichever choice we make is the one with the highest level of importance. It's that simple.

Here are common reasons and excuses people often use to put their healing on hold:

- Too much going on with kids' school activities.
- Moving to a new area.
- Waiting on a tax return.
- Big project at work.
- The economy isn't good.
- Going on vacation.
- Husband doesn't want to spend the money.
- Don't want to change my diet.
- Not interested in uncovering hidden emotional issues.

All this means is the move, the work project, the husband's opinion, or summer vacation is more important than getting healthy. Or it means that there isn't enough self-worth or belief that healing is possible. Again, this isn't a judgment, it's just a fact.

We choose the things that are most important to us, and our paradigm is the one making that decision.

When we say we want one thing (better health, calmer life, more happiness), but we continue to put other things ahead of those wants, that's telling the body, "Better heath, a calmer life, and more happiness aren't a priority."

Think of how that message impacts your energy vibration and gene expression. Imagine how your body will respond to get your attention and make you understand that it's in trouble and needs your help.

Chapter 29 – Identifying Hurdles To Healing

There is an old proverb that goes something like this: "If you don't have time to meditate for an hour every day, you should meditate for two hours." In other words, if you think you are too busy to do the thing that will help you, then you need even more help than you think.

Every message, every conversation, every belief in you right now is being compounded every second and influencing your trajectory positively or negatively. Every choice will either take you closer to your goals or further away from them.

If your patterns, thoughts, beliefs, and blocks stopping you do not shift, and you stay on your current health trajectory, what will your life look like in three years?

We've had clients who were literally given months to live, who turned their health and their lives completely around. It's because they believed healing was possible and they took action and followed the plan we created for them.

Ask yourself: "If I don't make this change today, where does that put me tomorrow? Can I wait three more weeks? Can I wait three more months? Can I wait three more years to get the support, tools, and healing I need?"

Your life today is a reflection of what you've experienced, believed, or thought to this point. Whatever you do, whatever you believe today will create your tomorrow. And your tomorrow will either be closer to your goals or further away. You get to choose which direction you go in.

Chapter Takeaways

- Whenever you make a decision to stick with the status quo rather than doing something that will change your life circumstances, it means your subconscious believes what you are experiencing currently is "safer" than doing something different.

- Choices are based on priorities. When you have choice, whichever one you choose over the other means you value that choice (or what you believe that choice will give you) more than what you think the other choice will give you. Period.

- Your life today is a reflection of everything you've thought, experienced, and believed. The only way to change what your life will look like tomorrow is to change something in your thoughts, actions, and beliefs right now.

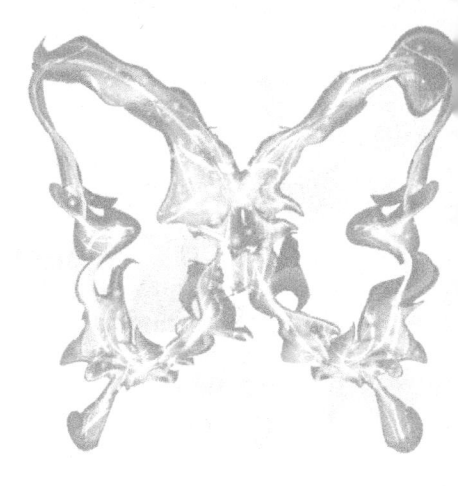

CHAPTER 30

DEFENSE MECHANISMS

We are wired to create defense mechanisms to protect ourselves against perceived danger. You hid the key to these defense mechanisms from yourself to stay safe. And since you hid the key from yourself, it's difficult to find the hiding place on your own.

The good news is:

As long as you have the belief and the willingness to step up and do what it takes to get yourself on the right health trajectory, and you work with a practitioner who believes the key is available and knows how to help you find the key, you not only can find it but also use it to move forward past your defense mechanisms.

The team here at Nourish is especially good at helping clients move past their hidden blocks and transform their health because each of us has gone through our own healing experience, we've done the work personally, and we've been working with clients for more than a decade helping them do it, too.

One of the reasons we can see through your defense mechanisms faster and more easily than you can is because you didn't design them for us to not be able to see past, you designed them for you not to see past, even when they are blatantly staring you in the face.

Here's what is most important to know:

You were designed to heal, and you already inherently have what you need to do that. You just may need some outside guidance to see what you're protecting yourself from seeing.

The most important question: *Is your desire to heal bigger than your fear of changing and moving beyond the blocks keeping you stuck on your current health trajectory?*

Because here's the blunt truth: If there is any reason you aren't moving forward right now to change your current health trajectory, that means that your paradigm is set to believe your current experience is "safer" than changing it.

And you might be arguing back at this book saying:

"No, no, no. Really. There's a real reason. It's not an excuse. I really don't have the time to focus on myself."

Or you might be thinking:

"Seriously. This is for real. I don't have the resources to do what I know I need to do to get healthier."

Or you're pushing back and saying:

"This isn't a defense mechanism. I swear, the reason I'm not prioritizing my health right now is because my kids (spouse, mother, aunt, boss) need me to help them, so I have to do that and can't spend the time and energy on myself."

If this is stirring you up right now, that's good! Because it means that you're tap dancing right on top of *the very thing that's been stopping you* from getting everything you say you want.

Any reason you have right now for not moving forward and taking action, is connected to an underlying hidden block in the way of your transformational healing experience. Period.

Again, that's not a judgment. Our paradigm only allows us to make choices we believe will help us, and does not allow us to take action on something we perceive as dangerous. But when you are aware of the block, you can consciously choose to over-ride it.

Here are some examples of what your paradigm may have categorized as dangerous:

- Putting yourself first, because your identity is anchored to helping everyone else.
- Spending time focused on your healing because what if you can't do it and you confirm your belief that you are destined to fail?
- Reversing your symptoms and illness because you're so used to "being sick" that you wouldn't know who you are if you were healthy.
- Spending money on yourself because that would mean you are "selfish."
- Asking for help because you are used to people never coming through for you and not supporting you.
- Stepping up for yourself, and letting your spouse (kids, friends, family, etc.) know how important it is to you to get the support you need.
- Believing that you don't have to do everything on your own.

Right now, you are spending your time on something that is not getting you the health and life goals you want. You're spending money on something that is taking away from your ability to heal. And though the people around you may need your help, they also do not want you to suffer in order to help them. If you continue to push yourself to the side and suffer in an effort to help others, what message is that sending to your body and to the people you love?

Again, if you do not change your trajectory, and shift your paradigm what will your health and life look like in five years? What would your future Self tell you to do *right now* to change your trajectory?

The future version of you who took action and became the ideal healthy you, what would she tell you now?

In this book, on our YouTube channel, and in our programs, you can find the how. But you have to bring the belief, the desire, and the willingness to take action and get out of your own way.

Let's look at an example of how a hidden block and underlying fear can stop healing.

"Horseback Riding Lessons Are More Important Than My Life" Story

Before we will accept anyone as a client, we meet with them to make sure it's the right fit. Our goal as a company is to help clients find true, long-term health. And if they aren't ready to put their healing first, or we feel our process isn't the right fit for them, then we don't invite them into the program.

It's important to us that:

1. The person is ready to heal and believes it's possible.
2. They are willing to show up for themselves and follow the process.
3. They are coachable and willing to ask for help when they feel stuck.
4. They are the right fit for the amazing supportive community of clients that we've built.

Kirstin recently met with a woman named Heather who's an esthetician. She began sobbing as she described how bad her symptoms were getting.

"I literally have nightmares about my children being at my funeral."

"That must feel awful," Kirstin said.

"It does. And I feel guilty all the time because my kids don't even know the healthy me. All they see is a mom who is sick and cannot spend time with them because I'm either sleeping, running around trying to do laundry and clean the house, or trying to squeeze in clients each day. Which is a whole other thing: my business is starting to fall apart because I just can't find the time or the energy to take care of my clients, and I keep canceling on them."

"I have to do something, or I'm afraid I'm going to die."

She said she was ready to put herself and her healing first. She said she would do anything that it took. Kirstin discussed with her a plan to heal. She said she was ready to start. She was excited to move forward.

Then she said, "But I just can't afford it because I can barely afford to pay for my daughter's horseback riding lessons."

If you look at what she's saying, what is her underlying driver? What's the block between what she says she wants (changing her health trajectory so she can get her energy and life back) to what she's choosing (paying for horseback riding lessons rather than investing in herself.)

It's probably much easier for you to see what's stopping her. Of course, she's stuck in the idea that she has to put her needs after the needs of others. That's part of her identity. The struggle, the pain, the frustration, and even her "inability to find the right solution" is part of her paradigm.

She told me, "I couldn't possibly tell my daughter she would have to stop her lessons. It would crush her."

Wouldn't losing her mom crush her more?

The riding lessons were twice the amount as the investment in the program. Heather wouldn't even entertain the idea of cutting the lessons back to free up the amount needed to invest in herself.

"Do I have your permission to coach you right now?" Kirstin asked.

And she said, "Yeah."

"What's worse, your daughter being potentially disappointed because her horseback riding lessons were cut back? Or for her not to have the energetic, happy, healthy mom you know you can be?"

And that's when the real problem revealed itself.

"Can you even see yourself being the energetic version of yourself that you described?" Kirstin asked.

And quietly, Heather said, "No."

And that's where she was stuck. She didn't believe she could change and reach health.

Here's a hack:

Whenever we say things like "I don't have the time... or I can't afford...," What that really means is that our subconscious is saying: "I believe spending my time, money, or effort on something else is more important." The need to protect our paradigm is so strong that we will make decisions over and over that support that paradigm even if they also hurt us and go directly against what we say we want.

When you ask for something, and you are given that very thing, but then you find a reason to reject it, that's your paradigm fighting to keep the status quo.

What subconscious belief could be stopping you from transformational healing? Take five minutes and quickly list out everything you can think of without judgement of the answers. Just keep writing and allow the answers to surface.

Here's another great example of how hidden blocks can contribute to illness:

Lexi's Story

Lexi was a high school student when she started working with us, and doing great in the program. After about six months, she was off all her medications, and her symptoms were nearly gone. When she went off to college, everything changed. Within a few weeks, she wasn't feeling good and her symptoms began resurfacing. Her energy shifted, and she tapped into an old story that "she would never get better."

She wasn't doing the assignments the coaches gave her, she was stuck in her story, and she was missing coaching appointments. Her mom said that she was having epic meltdowns and calling her at all hours of the night crying about how bad she felt.

So, I asked her, "What's really going on here?"

"I don't know!" she said.

"What if you did know? What benefit is there to this relapse and feeling so bad?"

"There are no benefits to this. I hate it!" she exclaimed.

"Okay. So, what if there were a benefit. What might it be?"

"I don't know. Maybe it's because if I'm not sick, I don't have an excuse to go back to my mom and get the support that I really want."

And there it was. In plain sight. The root cause of her relapse. Her paradigm had spoken, and it was saying:

"When I get support from my mom, I feel safe. So, if I'm not sick, then I can't get the support I've anchored to feeling safe. So, in order to feel safe, I have to be sick."

And her mom, feeling so responsible and guilty because Lexi had been diagnosed with autoimmune at seven years old, over-supported her when she was a child, trying to take away any ounce of discomfort or pain. But in doing so, she got caught in a cycle of codependency. She over-supported in an attempt to squash her feelings of guilt, and her daughter leaned

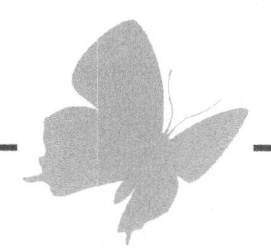

> Guilt and resentment go hand-in-hand. Where there is one, the other is present too, even if you don't see it immediately. Guilt is when you take on someone else's expectation and feel responsible if you don't meet that expectation. Resentment is when you project your expectations on someone else and are upset when that expectation isn't met. Where do you notice feelings of guilt? Where do you feel resentment? When you dissolve one, you will also dissolve the other.

into her symptoms to get the emotional support so she would feel better.

And then this cycle created resentment on both sides with each of them feeling frustration towards the other. Lexi was frustrated and resentful by the "hovering" when her mom tried to give support during times she didn't want it. Her mom was frustrated and resentful to Lexi for emotionally explosive episodes, demanding support.

To stop this unhealthy cycle, we worked with both of them to break the codependency, set boundaries for themselves and each other, clear the guilt and the resentment, and get on their own transformational healing trajectories. This allowed them to have an empathetic and supportive, yet not damaging relationship.

When we try to fix others, we take away their ability to learn and grow. And even though they may make a mistake or be challenged by the consequences of their behavior or choices, those experiences are important to their growth process. Understanding doesn't mean it's our role to fix them. Healing is a personal journey. Many of us have been conditioned to believe that love is caretaking, being "completed," or endlessly betraying ourselves to be chosen.

Healthy relationships allow each person the freedom to be themselves, without accepting abusive behavior, trying to fix the other person, or trying to become something you're not in an effort to be seen, accepted, or loved.

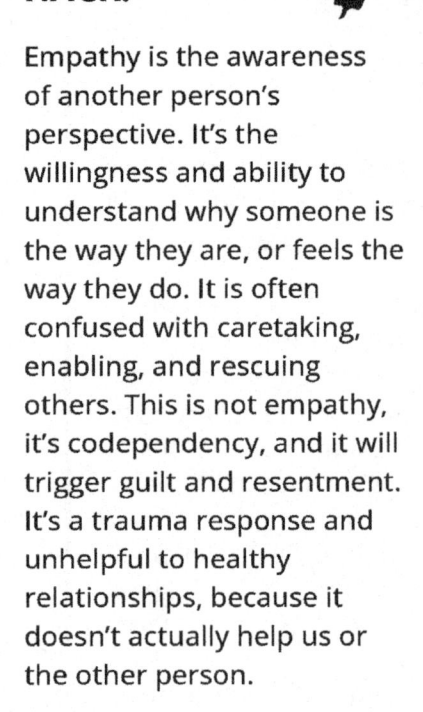

> **HACK:**
>
> Empathy is the awareness of another person's perspective. It's the willingness and ability to understand why someone is the way they are, or feels the way they do. It is often confused with caretaking, enabling, and rescuing others. This is not empathy, it's codependency, and it will trigger guilt and resentment. It's a trauma response and unhelpful to healthy relationships, because it doesn't actually help us or the other person.

Chapter Takeaways

- A defense mechanism is something you create to protect yourself from perceived danger, though it is difficult to identify and surface your own defense mechanisms because you hid the key to finding them from yourself to protect yourself from them.

- You were designed to heal, and you already have what you need to heal. You simply need the willingness and belief that healing is possible, along with the right support to guide you through the process.

- What are you focused on right now that may be preventing you from healing? Where do you perhaps see guilt, resentment, or codependency in your life that need to be dissolved?

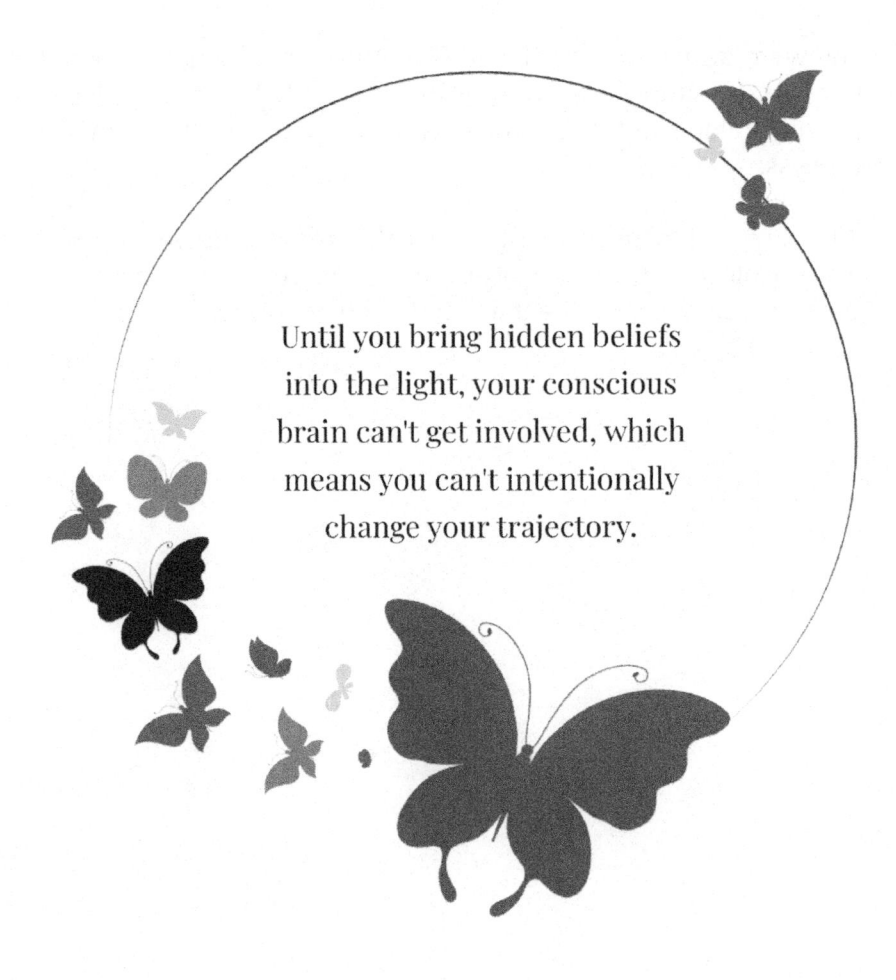

Until you bring hidden beliefs into the light, your conscious brain can't get involved, which means you can't intentionally change your trajectory.

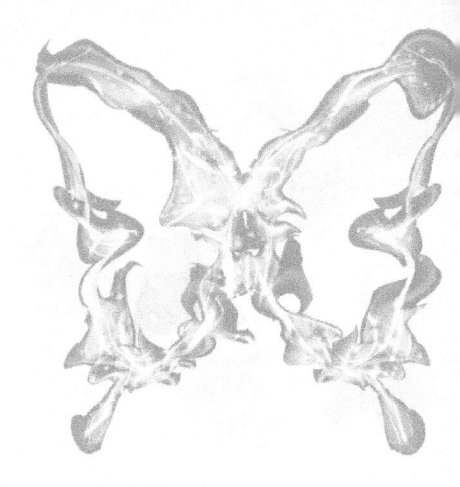

CHAPTER 31

CHANGING YOUR TRAJECTORY

Your paradigm in the hidden shadows of your subconscious drive your thoughts, decisions, and actions. One of the most important hacks to reaching the health goals that you've set for yourself, is to shine the light on those hidden beliefs and paradigms so your conscious mind can actually see them.

Until you bring hidden beliefs into the light, your conscious brain can't get involved, which means you can't intentionally change your trajectory.

We're going to show you a couple of the processes the Nourish Team uses with clients to help you rewire hidden blocks in your system, by bringing them out of the shadows, so your conscious brain (the one that actively makes change) can do something about them.

And then we're going to go even deeper so you can not only see this issue, but you can actually help reset the underlying pattern underneath it that's been keeping you stuck in a cycle of symptoms.

This is going to help you jump off the poor health trajectory onto the one that will lead you to transformational healing.

Are you up for these challenges?

Time Travel Exercise

There is a process we use with clients we call "time travel." It works with the subconscious wiring to surface past moments and change the perception of what happened in that moment. It can also allow clients to pull future moments into the now, though imagination and anchoring.

Though you can't change the past, you can change your perception of it and what your perception decides is "true."

What you perceive happened in any given moment is entirely based on who you were and the information you had, coupled with your life experiences up until that exact moment. You could only have done what you did in that moment, based on who you were at that point in time.

Many clients repeatedly beat themselves up for choices they made in the past. The reason they struggle is because they are looking at that past moment with the information, experience, and knowledge they have now. They judge themselves for not knowing what they know today, which of course, they couldn't possibly have had then. When they fully embrace the fact that they couldn't have done anything different in that past moment then they did, because the past version of them didn't have the same information they have today, they can dissolve their anger and guilt, and forgive that past version of themselves.

What you perceive in the moment to be true, is true in that moment. That perception will continue to be true until you alter the perspective. What you remember to be true in the past, is based on what version of you is looking at that moment. A judgmental version of you today, who feels guilt and shame will perceive the past differently than a balanced and grateful version of you today. It will also impact what you see in the future. Perception can change, and perception is in the eye of the beholder.

That is why five different people can experience the same moment but have different perceptions of truth to what happened. Each person's perception is based on the information they had going into that moment, which includes their traumas, life experiences, fears, expectations, and vision of the future. Each of those things will influence how each person experiences that moment, what they remember, and how it will shape their vision of the future.

Because the subconscious cannot tell the difference between a memory, a dream, a current experience, or a future vision. It balls them all up into one, not seeing time as linear.

The conscious brain sees time as linear and has to be involved to differentiate the past, present, dream, or vision of the future. The conscious brain has to be involved to change the perception of the memory, the interpretation of the dream, or the understanding of the image of the future vision.

This is important to understand, so you can rewire the blocks stopping you from healing. If a perception of a past experience is controlling your future vision, then you are going to struggle to change your trajectory.

This may stop you from launching that business you've always wanted to start. Or it may cause you to marry a "safe" but unexciting spouse even though your soul longs for passion, travel, and new experiences.

Your life today is a reflection of your perception of your past. And whatever you perceive, experience, or believe today is going to mold your future. Then tomorrow will be a reflection of everything that you've experienced, including the experience of today. Every moment can take you in a different direction.

If this scares you, take a deep breath. Really. Take a moment and breathe.

Knowing this should help empower you because now you realize you have the opportunity to change whatever happens from this moment forward. And **this moment is the only one you actually control. This one. Right now.**

Each day you get to add to the vision of what you want, or take away from it. It's why desire is so important. If you don't desire what you say you want, you won't reach it because you won't be willing to deal with whatever challenge is needed to break the pattern.

When we talk about "time travel," what that means is when you are consciously aware, you can "go back" and either change the perception of the past or "jump forward" to your vision of the future.

Stay with us here; if your perception of the past is controlling your decisions now and impacting how your future plays out, you can change your life by simply rewiring your perception.

Of course, we're not actually suggesting we can connect you with Marty McFly and Doc Brown from *Back to the Future* and send you racing back to your childhood in a souped-up DeLorean with a flux capacitor, but we are suggesting you can jump back to any moment you want and alter your perception of it, change your "truth," and impact your life now and forever.

Try this exercise:

List three moments when you felt you were either abandoned, shamed, controlled, fearful, or abused.

List at least ten details about each moment, making sure to include how you felt emotionally, what you experienced physically, and what you remember thinking at the time. List things such as:

- Who else witnessed this moment?
- What smells do you remember?
- What do you remember hearing?
- What other sensations (warm, cool, loud, quiet, open, closed, dry, damp) do you remember?
- What were you feeling emotionally?
- What were you feeling physically?
- What time of year/day was it?
- How old were you?
- What did the room or environment look like?

Look over the three moments you listed and choose the one that stands out the most to you.

- What was the dominating emotion of the moment you choose? (This is a great time to use the "Emotions Wheel" download from the resources webpage.)
- When was the first time, or earliest time you remember feeling that emotion?
- Who was involved in that early experience?

List ten more details about that earlier moment, making sure to include how you felt emotionally, what you experienced physically, and what you remember thinking at the time.

Take a deep breath.

Now imagine that you are moving away from the moment and are now watching that moment through a glass window about 25 feet away. Know with certainty that you are safe and cannot be harmed. You are your current adult Self with all the knowledge of your current Self.

As you look through the glass at that earlier moment:

- What do you see now about that moment that perhaps you didn't see at the time?
- What compassion do you perhaps now have for the past version of yourself?
- What understanding do you now perhaps have for anyone else in that past experience?
- Look around that moment, what else do you see or notice as you look through the glass, from a safe distance, from the eyes of an emotionally stable adult self?
- What do you notice about your perceived experience from that past moment that was perhaps skewed or uninformed?

Breathe deeply and purposefully.

Now, imagine yourself, knowing what you know now and the new information you've gained in this exercise, crouching down to meet the eye level of that earlier version of you and making eye contact with her. Hold her hands and tell her exactly what she needed to hear in that moment to feel seen, heard, and safe.

Breathe again deeply with intention knowing you are safe and exactly where you need to be.

Now imagine yourself floating away from that earlier moment and coming back in this current moment. How do you feel? What has shifted? What is different?

To access a guided audio version of this exercise, go to the added resources page at www.nourish123.com/thbonus

Notice over the next few days and weeks how your thoughts and actions may have shifted due to this exercise. Do you feel freer? Are you connecting better with yourself and seeing your past differently? Are your dreams or thoughts shifting?

Your imagination is powerful and it's what connects the past, present, and future together in one big ball in your subconscious. Use that to your advantage.

It's a process that you've most likely been doing without realizing it, but it may have been stopping you from reaching your goals and getting on the health trajectory you want.

SCAN ME!

To access a guided audio version of this exercise, go to the added resources page at www.nourish123.com/thbonus

Chapter Takeaways

- It is critical to uncover subconscious hidden beliefs and surface them so you can bring the conscious mind into the mix. Without the conscious awareness, you cannot change your trajectory and shift to transformational healing.

- The Rewire Exercise is incredibly helpful in shifting your trajectory and eliminating old patterns that will pull you back to what is familiar yet not necessarily healthy.

- The Time Travel Exercise was designed to help shift perspective of past experiences and change your current beliefs about those moments.

Removing Blocks to Reach Goals Exercise

Look at the top three goals from your answers in Chapter 1: Goals, and choose the one that calls to you the most.

Perhaps your top three goals were to lose weight, increase energy, and have a better relationship with your spouse. Choose one of those goals and make it as specific as you can and attach the reason why you want that goal.

For example, if your goal is to increase your energy, also attach the reason for wanting that energy to the goal.

- I want increased energy, so I can start my coaching business and see ten clients a week.
- I want increased energy, so I can interact with grandchildren twice a week for three hours a day.
- I want increased energy, so I can walk a minimum of 30 minutes a day around my neighborhood.

When you are specific with your goals, and you connect them to personally compelling reasons, it's easier to envision them, which increases your ability to achieve.

Can you see the goal? Can you literally see it? When you close your eyes are you able to imagine the version of you who has reached that goal? Take a few minutes to really see her. What is she feeling? What does her life look like? Who does she spend her time with? What is happening for her personally and professionally? What details are connected to her?

This future version of you needs to step in and help you through the challenges that will arise as you move towards the goal. The challenges that come with the pursuit of any goal are what stop most people from reaching them. **Knowing that every goal always comes with challenges will help you move past them. Willingness to move through a challenge is what separates a want from a desire.**

Be clear about what you want and don't say what you're "supposed to say."

Maybe rather than "I want to lose weight," what you really want is to feel more comfortable in my clothes.

Perhaps you want to feel better, climb the stairs more easily, fit into your favorite dress, or be able to breathe more deeply, and you know that the amount of extra weight that you're carrying is impeding all those things.

Though weight is one of the most common ways people measure "success," it's a terrible measure for true health. Create a goal that is easier to envision and compelling to you to reach. Imagining yourself "breathing more easily after climbing stairs" will influence your subconscious much more deeply than seeing a number on the scale.

Breathing and the ability to do it freely impacts your system emotionally, mentally, and physically and goes directly to feeling safe, which is exactly what we are hard wired to find.

Maybe losing weight isn't a goal for you. How about your relationship with your spouse or someone else important in your life? How long has it been since you were excited to be intimate with your spouse? Maybe you want to feel more patience with your family. Because if you're feeling frustrated and snapping at people, it's not about them. No matter how annoying they are, no matter what's going on, there's something within you that is being triggered and needs attention.

Maybe your goal is to feel more confident in yourself, so you can express yourself to your spouse more easily. Maybe he's not closed off, perhaps you're not expressing yourself, and you're really annoyed because he can't guess what you're thinking?

This frustration can turn to resentment because you feel like you can't talk to him. That frustration is really about you. Because even if it's 100% true that your spouse is not open to communicating with you, it's still about you. Why are you continuing to stay in that type of negative environment? If you feel like you are in a situation where no one hears you, and you feel invisible, you have to ask yourself: "Why am I attracting or staying around people who can't see me?"

Choose a goal, make it specific, and get clear on why is it important to you. If you don't know why it's important to you, you won't reach it because you aren't connected to your true desire for it.

Tapping into your true desire will help you achieve pretty much anything as long as you're willing to do what's necessary to get it. Desire drives willingness. When people don't reach their goals, it's typically because they say they want it, but they don't truly *desire* it.

Wanting something is often tied to what people think they're "supposed to" want based on conditioning from society, family, friends, and the media. It's why so many people reach goals like the big house, the corner office, the perfect family, or the fancy car, but feel unfulfilled when they achieve them.

Desire comes when we want something, understand why we want it, and are willing to work through the challenges that will come in the pursuit of getting it.

So, when you choose a goal, the most important part is understanding why you want it. Why do you desire having more energy? Why do you desire a better relationship with your spouse? Why do you desire losing weight? What is driving your choice of that goal?

The difference between want and desire will impact your ability to reach your goal and feel fulfilled when you achieve it.

Hardwired into the subconscious is the need to belong to "the tribe" because your chances of survival are higher when you are protected by a group. That's why the beliefs of a group, as we discussed in Chapter 14: The Immune System, are so influential to the choices people make. The subconscious need to stay safe is connected to what "the tribe" says is "right."

This is why shame, fear, and abandonment are such powerful emotional responses. They are directly tied to survival. If your true desire for something is in conflict with what the tribe wants for you, this triggers fear.

This is often at the core of family disputes and why people are desperate to "belong."

It's one of the most common root issues we see with clients struggling with autoimmune disease, heart disease, cancer, and related symptoms because they are living a life that may keep them safe in the tribe, but is in conflict with what they desire personally.

Trying to live somebody else's version of who we're supposed to be is traumatic. And unprocessed trauma impacts gene expression and triggers symptoms, illness, and disease.

To recap, here are the simplified steps to removing blocks keeping you from reaching a goal:

1. Choose a goal.
2. Be specific about the goal.
3. Include a compelling reason (the why) for wanting the goal.
4. Imagine the version of you who has reached the goal.
5. Get specific about the vision of your future Self so you can truly see, feel, and embody her.
6. Have that future you help your current you make decisions and take action until you reach the goal. (This is another way to utilize the Time Travel exercise, by bringing the future to the influence the now, and in turn, influence your future.)

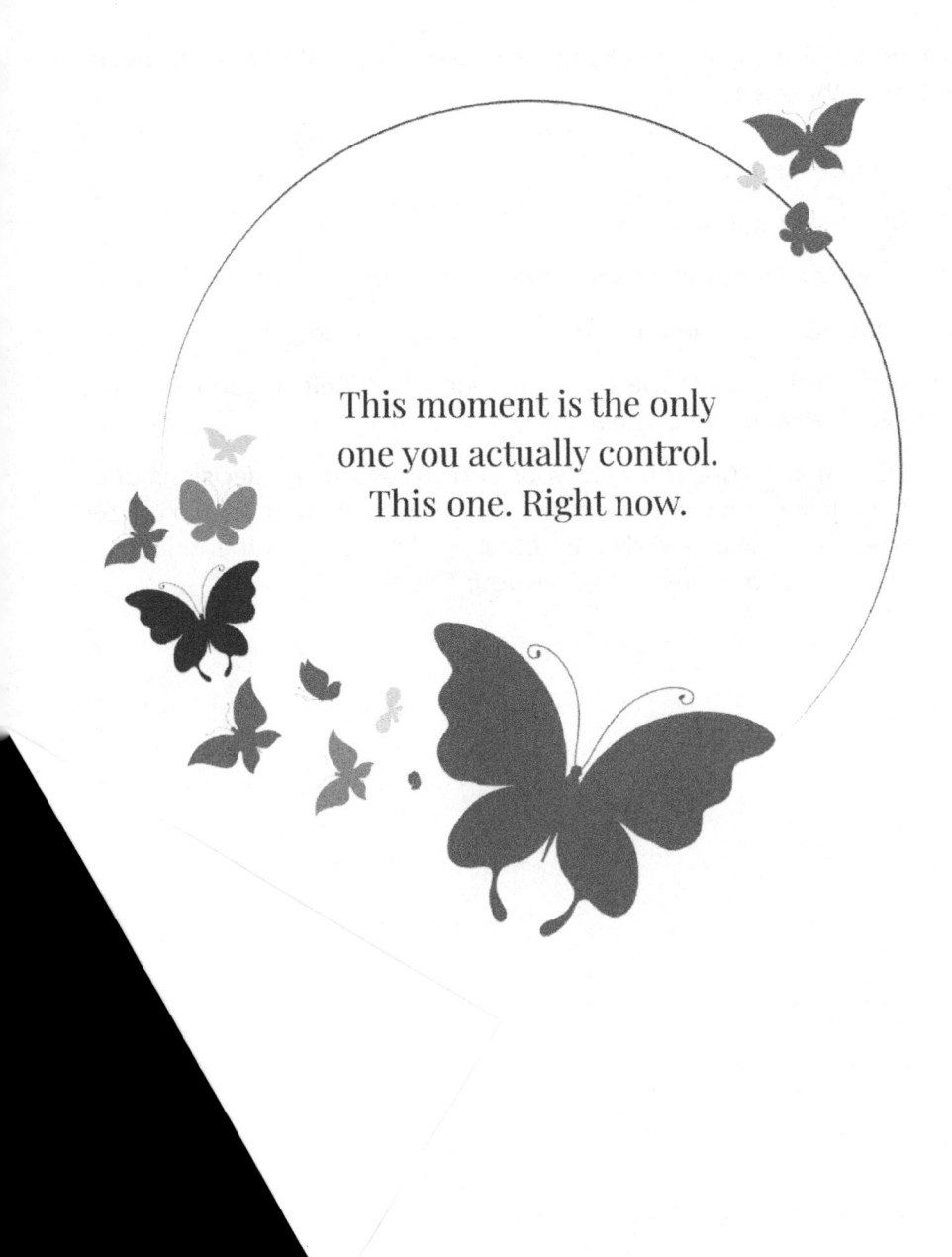

This moment is the only one you actually control. This one. Right now.

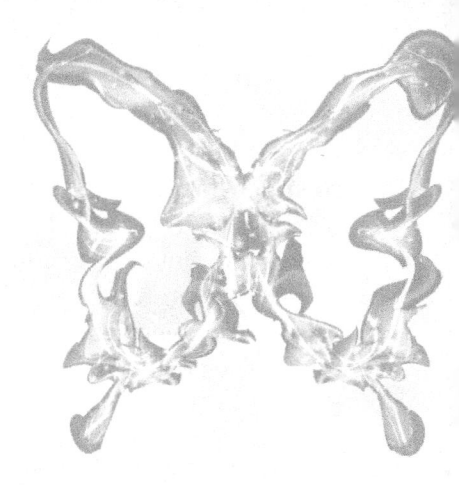

CHAPTER 32

THREE KINDS OF PEOPLE

As natural health practitioners, we've come across thousands of people who are struggling with symptoms and diagnoses. We've presented to support groups, been interviewed on podcasts, interacted with people at conferences, hosted dozens of healing events, and spoken directly with people who contact us to find out how they can work with us.

What we've found, and you've probably noticed this too, is that people typically fall into one of three categories:

The Struggle Person - This type of person has fully identified with their diagnosis or symptom. They join support groups on Facebook or local groups filled with people complaining about their symptoms. They discuss how people in their lives simply don't understand what they are going through. They share memes that reinforce the struggle of living with Hashimoto's, irritable bowel disease, PCOS, arthritis, chronic fatigue syndrome, insomnia, and anxiety. They are looking for people to connect with, commiserate with, and reinforce their experience. Though they complain about their condition, they aren't willing to make the changes necessary to heal. They aren't willing to change their diet, investigate underlying traumas, or alter their regular patterns in any way. They are more comfortable with their current experience and identify strongly with their situation, so they continue to repeat the patterns that cause their struggle. They say things like "I can't start the business I've always dreamed of because my Hashimoto's causes me so much fatigue." Or "My anxiety is so bad that I have to stay on disability because I can't go back to work." Or "I could never stop eating cheese, so that diet isn't going to work for me." They own the condition as part of who they are, which means the condition owns them. They are disempowered and disinterested in solutions that would eliminate their struggle, because the diagnosis is so much a part of who they are that they simply cannot see a life without it.

The Hidden Blocks Person - This type of person doesn't want to learn to "live with" their condition or health situation, they are looking for an answer to how to live without it. They know deep down that there has to be an answer, but they haven't yet found one. They have researched, read, and investigated. They've tried the diets, supplements, and recommendations found in their research, which have given them some limited success, but nothing that lasts long term. They may have even dipped their toe in alternative modalities like acupuncture, meditation, and therapy, but they are still stuck without a complete solution. There is often an underlying belief that they have to pull together all the pieces to the solution themselves and may feel like they are "failing" because they haven't yet "figured it out." They typically put the needs of others before their own, and won't invest the time, money, or effort in their personal journey because they don't feel worthy enough to do so. So, they continue to try to piece together a healing strategy with the resources they scrape together after everyone else has been taken care of. They feel guilty, they struggle with resentment, they feel frustrated, and they are exhausted. Even if they find the right solution, they won't allow themselves to take it because they can't let go of the feeling that they don't deserve it.

The Incomplete Puzzle Person - This person is positive there is a solution out there for them that includes the tools and support they need. Despite all the doctors they've seen, all the research they've done, and alternative therapies they've tried, they haven't come across the right strategy. They are tired, frustrated, and often feel misunderstood, but are willing to make their healing a priority. Though they might feel a little nervous, they are excited and ready to take on the challenges they know are part of the right healing solution. They are ready to invest the time, money, and commitment for themselves to get on the right path and reach the healing they are seeking. Their biggest issue is finding a cohesive solution with the right combination of pieces to create their unique healing puzzle. But when they do, they jump on it and dive in headfirst.

Not everyone was meant to heal, but everybody is capable of it. It doesn't matter why people are stuck in their personal health struggle. The most important thing is to recognize it is a struggle and to stop repeating the things that don't produce results. Complaining doesn't produce healing. Staying attached to the belief that you are sick and your current situation cannot change won't produce healing. And holding on to the false idea that you are not worth the investment of resources it takes to heal long term won't produce results.

Know there is a cohesive solution just for you. Because there is.

All you have to do is make the choice to put yourself first and grab the solution.

That alone, will make a difference in your health experience.

Chapter Takeaways

- There are three kinds of people who say they want a healing solution (The Struggle Person, The Hidden Blocks Person, and The Incomplete Puzzle Person), but typically, only one of them will achieve true healing transformation.

- Not everyone will find healing, though everyone is capable of it.

- There is a cohesive solution just for you. You simply need to grab it when it presents itself.

There is a cohesive solution just for you. All you have to do is make the choice to put yourself first and take action to grab that solution.

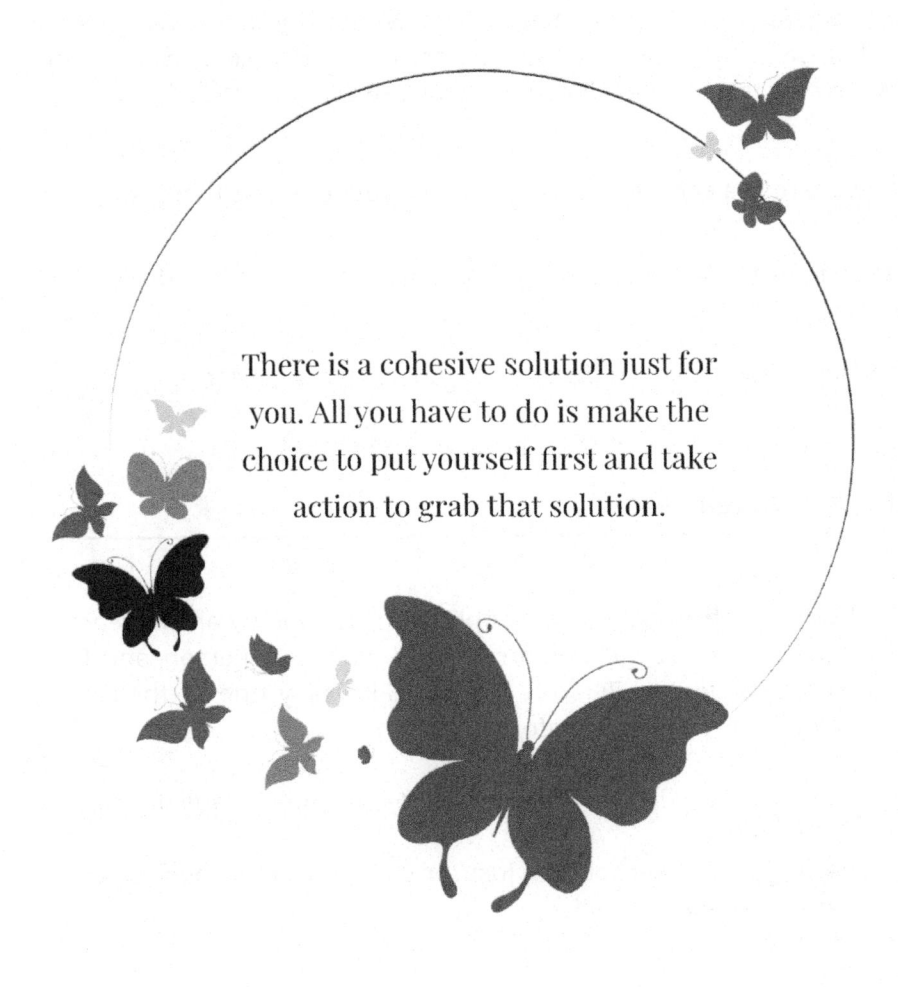

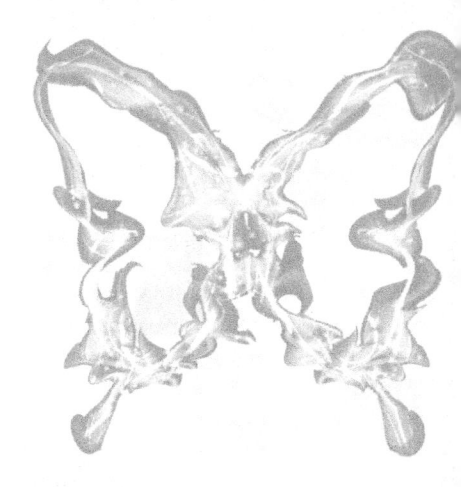

END:

TAKING ACTION AND FINDING YOUR FREEDOM

Now that you've read this book, and completed the exercises, you should have a clear understanding of your inherent power to directly influence your gene expression and live the life you desire. You now know how critical it is to have the Nutrition, Science, and Soul pieces dancing together synergistically so you can move onto your ideal health trajectory.

You also know that no matter what you've been told or what attempts you've made in the past, that healing is available to you.

Take a moment now, and imagine the transformed, healthy version of you.

Imagine the version of you who has *already achieved* your 12-week, 12-month, and 3-year health goals. "Time travel" and truly see the you that is living your ideal healthy life.

In that vision, what does your day include? With whom do you spend your time? What choices and actions do you make regularly with intention? What is your favorite place to vacation? Where are you living? What is it like to feel so empowered? How wonderful is it to connect with your Self and your core purpose? How different does your life look and feel in that future vision?

You can absolutely achieve that version of you. She's in there, waiting to get out.

You are an everyday miracle. And the miracle version of you is excited to present herself to the world. All you have to do is take action and let her shine through.

What are you waiting for?

Perhaps we'll get to tell your story at the beginning of our next book!

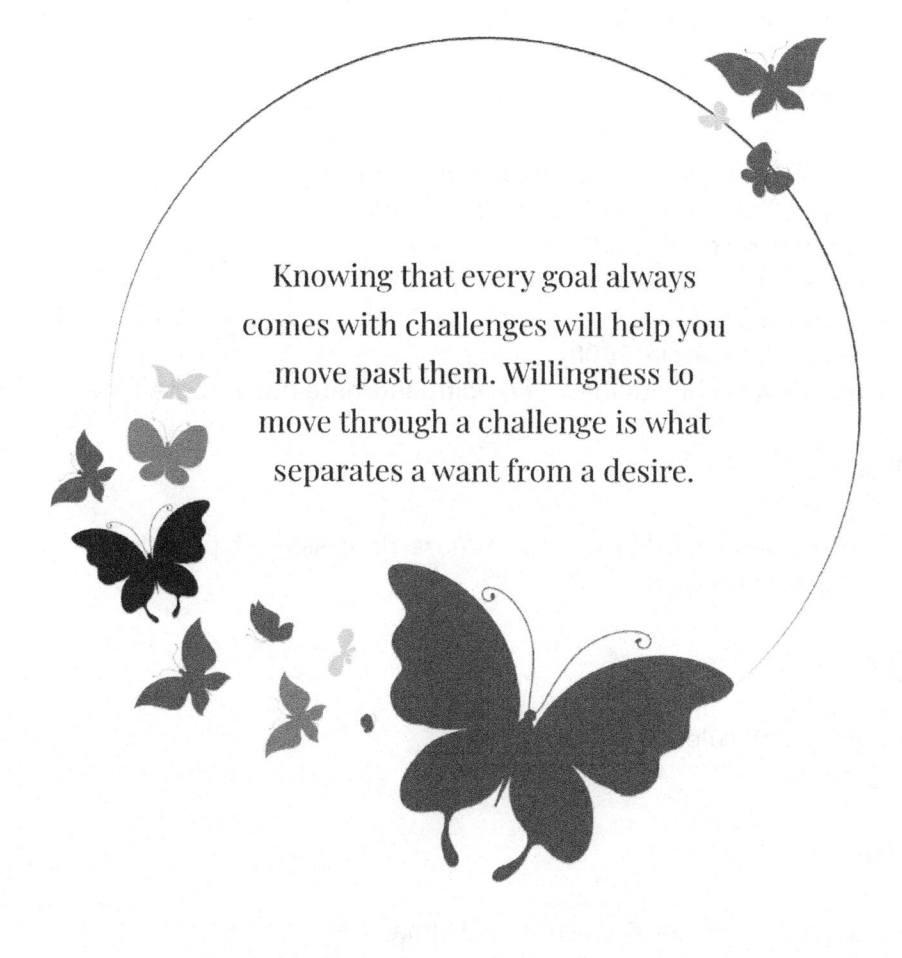

Knowing that every goal always comes with challenges will help you move past them. Willingness to move through a challenge is what separates a want from a desire.

ENDNOTES

Chapter 9

1. J. Tips, S. Cernohous, The Microbial Alliance - Friends & Foes in Life's Greatest Contest. (AppleADayPress 2014), pp. 22.
2. https://www.ncbi.nlm.nih.gov/pmc/articles/PMC1470005/

Chapter 11

1. https://ehe.health/blog/restorative-movement/
2. https://finnishwellbeing.com/en/restorative-movement-to-support-recovery-and-stress-management/
3. https://dynamicmedicalfitness.com/blog/restorative-exercises
4. S. Saraswati, Asana Pranayama Mudra Bandha. (Yoga Publications Trust, Bihar, India, 2008).
5. https://www.healthline.com/health/alternate-nostril-breathing

Chapter 12

1. https://www.bioinformant.com/hazardous-sleep-deprivation-affects-stem-cells/

Chapter 13

1. Pert, Molecules of Emotion.
2. Ibid.

Chapter 14

1. Steve Cole: Social Regulation of Human Gene Expression, UCLA

Chapter 15

1. D. Weatherby, S. Ferguson, Blood Chemistry and CBC Analysis: Clinical Laboratory Testing from a Functional Perspective. (Bear Mountain Publishing 2002), p. xi.

Chapter 17

1. https://ethics.harvard.edu/blog/new-prescription-drugs-major-health-risk-few-offsetting-advantages
2. M. Pollan, In Defense of Food: An Eater's Manifesto, 2008 Audiobook.

Chapter 18

1. B. Diaz and K. Ressler, "Parental Olfactory Experience Influences Behavior and Neural Structure in Subsequent Generations," Nature Neuroscience 17, no. 1 (January 2014), pp. 89-96.
2. L. Rankin, The Fear Cure, Cultivating Courage as Medicine for the Body, Mind and Soul. (Hay House, Inc. 2015), p. 64.

IMPLEMENT WHAT YOU'VE LEARNED

12 Week Healing Success

GUIDEBOOK PLANNER

Looking for help implement what you've learned in this book over the next 12 weeks?

Grab a copy of the Transformational Healing Guidebook Success Planner.

www.nourish123.com/thbonus

SCAN ME!

Nourish Transformational Healing Programs

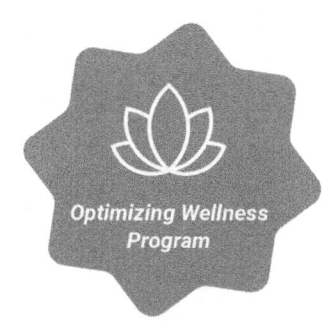

Optimizing Wellness Program

1. **Optimizing Wellness** - For people who are sliding off their ideal health trajectory and want to get back on the right path before issues turn into disease.

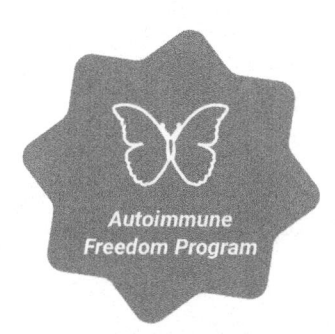

Autoimmune Freedom Program

2. **Autoimmune Freedom Program** - For people who want to get out of health crisis and into healing. They may or may not have an "official" diagnosis, but typically have been struggling with symptoms and chronic issues for several years, and are ready for a customized solution.

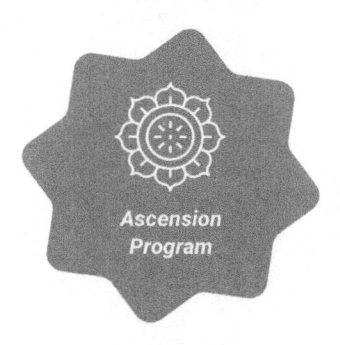

Ascension Program

3. **Ascension Program** - For people who have transformed out of crisis and into healing, and are ready for an advanced level of transformation physically, mentally, emotionally, and spiritually so they can reach their full potential.

To learn more about our programs and how we might be able to help you, book a call with the Nourish team:

www.nourish123.com/heal

AMAZON REVIEW REQUEST

Thank You for Reading Our Book!

We really appreciate all of your feedback and
we love hearing what you have to say.

We need your input to make the next version of
this book and our future books better.

Please take two minutes now to leave a helpful review
on Amazon letting us know what you thought of the book:

www.nourish123.com/bookreview

Thanks so much!

- Kirstin and Anthony

Thank you

P.S. If you found this book helpful, and especially if you've had
success implementing the content in these pages, please leave a
review on Amazon letting us know your story.

VERY NEXT STEPS

Book a call with the Nourish team
if you're ready to get started
with your health and you'd like our help:
www.nourish123.com/heal

SPECIAL THANKS

Every now and then, people who come into your life who create an impact that changes the flow of your life in a way that cannot be appropriately explained in words. It must be felt. Our clients are those people. And so is our entire team.

We want to especially point out that the publication of this book, the guidebook, and the additional resources were only possible because of the dedication, brilliance, and support of:

Briana Boldin - who is a wizard when it comes managing Operations and Client Experience. Her ability to see the big picture and pay attention to detail is remarkable. She keeps us doing what we do best. Thank you!

Jessica Pavone - who jumped into handling the social media, advertising, and marketing with both feet beautifully so we could present the most amazing product possible. Thank you!

Jeremy Kenerson and DeskTeam360. So much gratitude. So so much!

Made in the USA
Middletown, DE
12 January 2024